CARB CYCLING DIET 2024

120 Recipes Advanced Nutritional Strategies The Ultimate Method to Lose Weight Without Giving Up Carbohydrates

TERY LONG

DISCLAIMER

This book aims to provide useful and informative material on the topics covered in the publication. It is sold with the understanding that the author and publisher are not engaged in rendering any personal medical, health care, or other professional services in the book. The reader should consult his or her physician, health care provider, or other competent professional before adopting any suggestions in this book or drawing any conclusions. The author and publisher expressly disclaim any responsibility for any liability, loss, or risk, personal or otherwise, arising, directly or indirectly, from the use and application of any contents of this book.

NOTE FOR THE MUG

In the context of this book, when we refer to "a cup" as a unit of measurement for ingredients, we mean using a standard kitchen cup with a capacity of approximately 240 milliliters. It is essential to use a measuring cup to get the right quantities of ingredients. If you don't have a measuring cup, you can use a graduated measuring cup, making sure to correctly correspond to the proportions indicated. Here are some examples 1 Cup of flour 100 gr. 1 cup of rice 200 gr. 1 Cup of Quinoa 200 g, It is recommended to level the dry ingredients in the cup using a spatula or the blade of a knife to obtain an accurate measurement. For liquid ingredients it is recommended to fill the cup to the brim without squeezing or leaving gaps. However, it is important to keep in mind that ingredient measurements may vary.

RECIPES APPETIZERS

85 GRILLED PRAWN SKEWERS

87 GUACAMOLE WITH ZUCCHINI CHIPS

89 BOILED QUAIL EGGS WITH SALT AND PEPPER

91 CHEESE BALLS WITH WALNUTS

93 BRUSCHETTE WITH TOMATO AND BASIL ON WHOLEMEAL BREAD

95 CROSTINI WITH HUMMUS AND DRIED TOMATOES

97 CHICKEN MEATBALLS WITH BBQ SAUCE

99 POTATO SALAD WITH GREEK YOGURT AND MUSTARD

101 CHICKEN WRAPS WITH GRILLED VEGETABLES

104 SWEET POTATO NACHOS WITH AVOCADO SAUCE

107 QUINOA SALAD WITH ROASTED VEGETABLES

110 SMOKED SALMON ROLLS WITH CHEESE

112 CHICKPEA MEATBALLS WITH YOGURT SAUCE

RECIPES FIRST DISHES

140 WHOLEMEAL RISOTTO WITH MUSHROOMS AND SPINACH

142 WHOLEMEAL PASTA WITH COURGETTES AND SMOKED SALMON

144 ZUCCHINI SPAGHETTI WITH CHICKEN MEATBALLS

146 SHRIMP AND AVOCADO SALAD WITH LIME SAUCE

148 EGG OMELETE WITH SPINACH AND CHEESE

150 ZUCCHINI SPAGHETTI WITH GARLIC BUTTER SAUCE

152 BAKED SALMON ON A BED OF SPINACH

154 CARPACCIO OF ZUCCHINI WITH DRIED TOMATOES AND CHEESE

156 GHERKIN PAD THAI WITH GRILLED CHICKEN

158 GRILLED AUBERGINES WITH TOMATO PESTO

160 COURGETTE LASAGNE WITH RICOTTA AND MEAT SAUCE

162 PORCINI MUSHROOM RISOTTO WITH PARMESAN

165 CHICKEN SALAD WITH AVOCADO AND VEGETABLES

167 BROWN RICE SPAGHETTI WITH ARUGULA PESTO

169 SWEET POTATO OMELETTE WITH BACON AND ONION

172 POTATO GNOCCHI WITH TOMATO SAUCE

174 ZUCCHINI TAGLIATELLE WITH LIGHT ALFREDO SAUCE

176 QUINOA RISOTTO WITH ASPARAGUS AND CHEESE

178 ZUCCHINI SPAGHETTI WITH LEMON PRAWNS

180 GRILLED SALMON WITH CAULIFLOWER RISOTTO

183 WHOLE WHOLE SPAGHETTI WITH FRESH TOMATO SAUCE

185 PASTA SALAD WITH GRILLED VEGETABLES

187 SPELLED RISOTTO WITH MUSHROOMS AND PARMESAN

189 CHICKEN CACCIATORA WITH WHOLE BARLEY

192 WHOLE WHOLE PAPPARDELLE WITH BOLOGNESE SAUCE

195 QUINOA SALAD WITH CHICKPEAS AND PEPPERS

197 BUCKWHEAT SPAGHETTI WITH SPINACH PESTO

199 BARLEY RISOTTO WITH COURGETTES AND PEPPERS

201 EGG OMELETATE WITH BACON AND POTATOES

203 LENTIL SPAGHETTI WITH TOMATO SAUCE

205 PIZZA WITH CAULIFLOWER CRUST

207 AUBERGINES LASAGNE WITH RICOTTA AND SPINACH

210 PUMPKIN GNOCCHI WITH BUTTER AND SAGE

RECIPES SECOND DISHES

235 TURKEY BREAST STUFFED WITH SPINACH AND CHEESE

237 CHICKEN MEATBALLS WITH TOMATO SAUCE

240 GRILLED TUNA WITH BLACK OLIVE SAUCE

242 PORK CURRY WITH BROCCOLI

244 CHICKEN WITH CASHEW SAUCE AND VEGETABLES

246 SALMON STEAK WITH PESTO SAUCE

248 GRILLED LAMB RIBS WITH MINT SAUCE

250 EGG OMELETTE WITH BACON AND MUSHROOMS

252 ROSEMARY CHICKEN WHITE WINE SAUCE

254 SPICY PRAWNS WITH CHILI SAUCE

256 FRIED TOFU WITH VEGETABLES AND SOY SAUCE

258 CHICKEN PARMESAN WITH WHOLE WHOLE PASTA

261 BAKED PORK STEAK WITH SWEET POTATOES

263 SALMON IN PAPER WITH BARLEY RISOTTO

266 CHICKEN CACCIATORA WITH POLENTA

269 TROUT FILLET WITH QUINOA AND VEGETABLES

271 BEEF STEAK WITH CAULIFLOWER PUREE

273 EGG OMELETATE WITH BACON AND POTATOES

2276 CHICKEN CURRY WITH BROWN RICE

278 FRENCH SOLE WITH MUSHROOM RISOTTO

281 MUSTARD PORK WITH CARROT PURE

283 PRAWNS IN COCONUT CREAM WITH ZOODLES

286 PULLED PORK WITH CALES SALAD

289 SESAME CHICKEN WITH STEAMED BROCCOLI

291 GRILLED SALMON WITH ALMOND BUTTER SAUCE

293 GRILLED TUNA WITH AVOCADO SAUCE

INTRODUCTION WHAT IS THE CARB CYCLING DIET

Carb Cycling Diet: The Ultimate Way to Lose Weight, Increase Energy, and Transform Your Body Without Giving Up Carbs Description: Have you ever wanted a way to enjoy carbs without compromising your weight loss or fitness goals? Have you ever wondered if there is a method that can offer you the best of both worlds: the pleasure of eating and the satisfaction of obtaining concrete results? Welcome to the world of Carb Cycling. "Carb Cycling Diet is your essential guide to understanding and mastering one of the most effective and sustainable nutritional strategies in the world of health and fitness. This diet is not a fad, but a proven approach that allows you to reap the benefits of carbohydrates at the right moments, while you burn

fat and build muscle. What you will find in this book: Detailed and Simple Introduction: You will learn what Carb Cycling is, how it works and why it is considered a well-kept secret by athletes and nutritionists. Personalized Meal Plans: You'll discover how to tailor Carb Cycling to your specific needs, whether you want to lose weight, gain muscle mass or simply improve your overall health. Tasty, Easy-to-Prepare Recipes: Enjoy delicious, nutritious meals that will keep you full and satisfied while meeting your dietary goals. Strategies for Long-Term Success: You'll learn to track your progress, overcome common obstacles, and stay motivated even on the toughest days. Be inspired by the experiences of those who have transformed their lives thanks to Carb Cycling.

This book is perfect for anyone who wants to start their journey to a healthier, stronger body, without having to give up the foods they love. It doesn't matter if you're a complete beginner or if you've tried other diets in the past, "Carb Cycling Diet will provide you with the tools and knowledge you need to achieve real, lasting results. Find out how Carb Cycling can transform the way you look at nutrition and fitness, helping you achieve your goals in a healthy, balanced and satisfying way. Get ready to transform your body and your life one carbohydrate at a time!

THE FUNDAMENTAL PRINCIPLES

The Fundamental Principles of Carb Cycling, How Carb Cycling Works Carb Cycling is a dietary strategy that is based on alternating carbohydrate intake on the days of the week to optimize body composition and improve physical performance. But how exactly does it work? The key concept of Carb Cycling is to adapt carbohydrate intake based on the body's energy and metabolic needs. High Carbohydrate Days: During these days, carbohydrate intake is high. These days are generally scheduled to coincide with intense training sessions or particularly demanding physical activity. The increase in carbohydrates allows you to replenish muscle glycogen reserves, ensuring sufficient energy to support physical activity and promote muscle growth.

Carbohydrates are used to fuel muscles and prevent protein breakdown, helping to maintain lean muscle mass. which helps reduce body fat. These days are often combined with less intense training sessions or rest days, when the body's energy demands are lower. Moderate Days: Some Carb Cycling plans also include days with a moderate carbohydrate intake. These days offer a balance of high and low carb, keeping energy stable without excess or deficiency. Moderate days are ideal for maintenance and to avoid extreme fluctuations in energy and hunger levels. This strategic alternation allows you to maximize the benefits of carbohydrates when they are most needed and minimize fat accumulation when they are not.

Furthermore, Carb Cycling can help keep your metabolism active, preventing the slowdown typical of restrictive diets, and offering greater flexibility than other diets, making it more sustainable in the long term. This explanation provides the reader with a clear understanding of how Carb Cycling works and why this strategy is effective for weight management and improving physical performance.

BENEFITS OF THE CARB CYCLING DIET

Carb cycling offers a series of benefits that make it an effective and attractive nutritional approach both for those who want to lose weight and for those looking to improve their athletic performance or maintain a toned and healthy physique. Below, we look at the main benefits of this diet: 1. Weight Loss and Body Fat Reduction One of the main reasons why many people choose Carb Cycling is its effectiveness in promoting weight loss and body fat reduction. By alternating high- and low-carb days, the body is encouraged to burn fat stores as an energy source, especially on low-carb days. This approach allows you to reduce fat without sacrificing muscle mass, which is often a problem in restrictive diets.

2. Maintenance and Growth of Muscle Mass
Unlike traditional low-carb diets, Carb Cycling allows you to maintain and even increase muscle mass. On high-carb days, the body receives the energy it needs to sustain intense workouts, promoting protein synthesis and muscle growth. This is especially important for athletes, bodybuilders and anyone who wants a more defined and toned physique. **3. Increased Energy and Athletic Performance** Carb Cycling allows you to maximize athletic performance thanks to the strategic intake of carbohydrates. On intense training days, the high carbohydrate content provides the energy needed to improve performance, allowing you to train with greater intensity and for longer periods. This not only helps you achieve better results, but also prevents the fatigue and burnout associated with overly restrictive diets. **4. Flexibility and Sustainability** One

One of the great advantages of Carb Cycling is its flexibility. Unlike many diets that require rigid and continuous restrictions, Carb Cycling allows you to vary your calorie and carbohydrate intake based on your personal needs and specific goals. This flexibility makes the diet easier to stick to in the long term, reducing the chance of feeling deprived or unmotivated.5. Metabolism Support and Plateau Prevention Carb Cycling helps keep the metabolism active, avoiding the slowdown that often occurs in prolonged low-calorie diets. By alternating high- and low-carb days, you keep your body in a constant state of "surprise," preventing metabolic plateaus and continuing to promote weight loss and your desired body composition. 6. Improved Insulin Sensitivity Varying carbohydrate intake in Carb Cycling can improve insulin sensitivity, helping you better manage blood sugar levels.

On low-carb days, the body becomes more efficient at using insulin, while on high-carb days, insulin helps replenish glycogen stores without causing excessive blood sugar spikes. These benefits demonstrate how the Carb Cycling Diet can be a powerful and versatile approach to improving health, body composition and physical performance. Readers who adopt this nutritional strategy can expect tangible results while maintaining a balanced and sustainable diet.

THE DIFFERENT APPROACHES TO CARB CYCLING

Carb cycling is not a one-size-fits-all diet plan; it is a flexible strategy that can be adapted to different goals, whether it is weight loss, increased muscle mass or improved athletic performance. Let's see how Carb Cycling can be customized for each of these purposes. Carb Cycling for Weight Loss Carb cycling is highly effective for those looking to lose weight, especially by reducing body fat. In this approach, the goal is to create a calorie deficit while maintaining an active and sustainable metabolism. Low-Carb Days: Most of the week is dedicated to low-carb days, which promote fat burning as your primary source of energy.

During these days, insulin, the hormone that facilitates fat accumulation, is reduced and the body is encouraged to use stored fat reserves. High-Carb Days: A few days a week are designated as high-carb days to replenish glycogen stores and prevent metabolic slowing, which is common in long-term diets. These days also help maintain muscle mass, which is essential for healthy, sustainable weight loss. Carb Cycling for Increased Muscle Mass Those looking to increase muscle mass find Carb Cycling a precious ally, as this strategy allows you to fuel your muscles with carbohydrates when they need them most, promoting growth and recovery. High Carb Days: Most of the week, particularly on weight training days, will feature a high carbohydrate intake. This provides the muscles with the energy they need tackle intense workouts and promotes protein synthesis, which is essential for muscle growth. Low Carb Days: Also for building muscle mass, there are some low carb days, generally during rest or light training days. This helps maintain a balanced calorie balance and avoid excessive fat accumulation during the muscle building phase. Carb Cycling for Athletic Performance For athletes, Carb Cycling can be customized to maximize sports performance, ensuring constant and sustainable energy without compromising body composition. High Carbohydrate Days: Athletes will have a high carbohydrate intake on more intense training days or close to competition. This ensures that glycogen stores are full, providing the energy needed for performance optimal and preventing muscle fatigue. Low Carb Days: On less intense training or recovery days, carbohydrate intake is reduced. This not only helps you maintain your weight and desired body composition, but it can also improve insulin sensitivity, optimizing carbohydrate utilization on high-carb days. These approaches demonstrate how carb cycling can be tailored to achieve specific goals, whether it's losing weight, gaining muscle mass or improving athletic performance. Each method is designed to make the most of the benefits of carbohydrates, while keeping the body in a state of balance and optimization.

CONCLUSION OF THE KEY POINTS AND FUTURE

Summary of Key Points Throughout this book, we have thoroughly explored the concept of Carb Cycling and how this nutritional strategy can be used to achieve a variety of goals, whether it be losing weight, gaining muscle mass, or improving athletic performance . We have seen that Carb Cycling: Optimizes the use of carbohydrates on intense training days, increasing energy reserves and improving performance. Promotes fat burning on low carb days, facilitating weight loss and muscle definition. It improves the flexibility and sustainability of the diet, adapting to personal needs and making it easier to maintain long-term results. Supports muscle growth and

prevention of loss of lean mass, thanks to the synchronization of carbohydrate intake with physical activity. How to Integrate Carb Cycling into Your Lifestyle Integrating carb cycling into your daily life doesn't have to be complicated. Here are some practical steps to get you started: Evaluate your goals: Before you start, clarify your main goals: lose weight, gain muscle mass or improve athletic performance. This will help you choose the most suitable Carb Cycling plan. Plan your meals: Organize your week based on your activities and divide the days into high, low and moderate carbohydrate intake. Planning your meals in advance will help you stick to the plan and optimize your results. Be flexible: While planning is important, maintaining some flexibility is essential. If your needs or schedule change, adjust your high or low carb days accordingly. Track progress: Track your results regularly to understand what works best for you. Make changes to the plan based on your progress and feedback from your body. Tips for the Future As you dive into the world of Carb Cycling, remember that every body is unique, and what works for one person may not be ideal for another. Here are some tips for the future: Experiment and adapt: Don't be afraid to experiment with different frequencies and amounts of carbohydrates to find the approach that works best for you. Carb cycling is a versatile strategy, and the key to success is customization. Maintain Balance: Although carbohydrates play a central role in Carb Cycling, don't forget the importance of a balanced diet that includes proteins, healthy fats, vitamins and minerals. Don't Neglect Recovery: Make sure you give your body the time it needs to recover, especially on low-carb days.

Rest and recovery are essential for muscle regeneration and overall well-being. Take advantage of the knowledge you gain: Now that you have a solid understanding of Carb Cycling, apply these principles not only to your diet, but also to other aspects of your life. A flexible and personalized approach can bring lasting benefits to health, fitness and overall well-being. This conclusion summarizes the main concepts of the book, offering the reader a clear path on how to integrate Carb Cycling into their lifestyle and providing practical suggestions for continuing to improve and adapt the strategy over time.

BREAKFAST RECIPES

35

COCONUT AND BANANA PROTEIN PANCAKES

Preparation time: 15 minutes

Cooking time: 10 minutes

Servings: 4

Ingredients

2 ripe bananas

100 g of oat flour

2 eggs

50ml of coconut milk

1 teaspoon baking powder

1 pinch of salt

Coconut oil to grease the pan

Preparation

Mash the bananas with a fork. In a bowl, mix the oat flour, baking powder and salt. Add the eggs, coconut milk and mashed bananas. Mix until you obtain a homogeneous mixture. Heat a non-stick pan and grease it with coconut oil. Pour a ladle of mixture into the pan and cook the pancakes for about 2-3 minutes on each side, or until golden brown. Tips You can add dried fruit or seeds for a crunchy touch.

ENERGIZING GREEN SMOOTHIE WITH SPINACH AND AVOCADO

Preparation of ingredients: 5-10 minutes

Blending: 1-2 minutes

Total time: 6-12 minutes

Ingredients:

1 ripe avocado

1 bunch of fresh spinach

1 banana

1/2 green apple

Juice of half a lemon

1 cup water or plant-based milk (almond, coconut)

Ice (optional)

Chia or flax seeds (optional)

Preparation:

Wash and prepare the ingredients: Wash the spinach and apple well. Peel the banana and avocado. Blend everything: Place all the ingredients in the blender and blend until smooth and homogeneous. If you want a thicker consistency, add less liquid. Serve: Pour your smoothie into a glass and garnish with a few leaves of fresh mint or chia seeds.Variations: For a sweeter taste: Add a date, a date or a spoonful of honey. For an exotic touch: Add a piece of pineapple or mango. grated or a pinch of turmeric. Benefits of this smoothie: Rich in vitamins and minerals: Spinach is an excellent source of iron, calcium and vitamin K, while avocado is rich in good fats and vitamin E. Source of fibre: The fiber contained in spinach and banana they aid digestion and give a feeling of satiety.

EGG WHITE OMELETTE WITH SPINACH AND CHERRY TOMATOES

Preparation time: 15 minutes

Cooking time: 15 minutes

Servings: 2

Ingredients

4 egg whites

100g of fresh spinach

50g of cherry tomatoes

20g of grated parmesan

1 clove of garlic

Salt and pepper to taste

Extra virgin olive oil to taste

Preparation

Wash and cut the spinach and cherry tomatoes. Fry the garlic in a pan with a drizzle of oil, then add the spinach and let it soften. In a bowl, beat the egg whites with a fork, adding salt and pepper. Pour the egg white mixture into the pan with the vegetables, add the cherry tomatoes and parmesan. Cook over low heat, covered, until the omelette is cooked. Tips You can customize the omelette by adding other vegetables, such as mushrooms or peppers. Serve hot or cold.

OAT AND CHIA SEED PORRIDGE WITH BERRIES

Preparation time: 5 minutes

Cooking time: 5 minutes

Servings: 1

Ingredients

50g of oat flakes

1 tablespoon chia seeds

250ml of milk (vegetable or cow's milk)

100g of mixed berries

1 teaspoon honey (optional)

Cinnamon powder to taste

Preparation

In a bowl, mix the oats, chia seeds and milk.
Place the bowl in the microwave for 2-3
minutes, or in a saucepan on the stove until
the porridge is creamy. Add the berries,
honey and cinnamon. Mix well. Tips You can
add dried fruit or seeds for a crunchy touch.
If you prefer a thicker porridge, add less
milk.

WHOLEMEAL TOAST WITH AVOCADO AND POACHED EGG

Preparation time: 10 minutes

Cooking time: 5 minutes

(toast) + 3-4 minutes (egg)

Servings: 2

Ingredients

2 slice of wholemeal bread

1 ripe avocado

2 eggs

White vinegar

Salt and freshly ground black pepper

Extra virgin olive oil

Preparation

Toast the bread: Heat a non-stick pan and toast the bread on both sides. Prepare the poached egg: In a saucepan, bring plenty of salted water to the boil with a spoonful of white vinegar. Gently crack the egg into a small bowl and pour it into the boiling water. Cook for 3-4 minutes, until the egg white is set. Prepare the avocado: Cut the avocado in half, remove the stone and peel the pulp. Mash it lightly with a fork. Assemble the toast: Place the mashed avocado on the toasted toast. Gently place the poached egg on top of the avocado. Season with salt, freshly ground black pepper and a drizzle of extra virgin olive oil. Tips You can add other seasonings to taste, such as sesame seeds, flax seeds or chili flakes.

ALMOND FLOUR AND BLUEBERRY MUFFINS

Preparation time: 20 minutes

Cooking time: 20-25 minutes

Servings: 6-8

Ingredients

100g of almond flour

50g of coconut flour

3 eggs

50g of erythritol (or other natural sweetener)

1 teaspoon baking powder

1/2 teaspoon baking soda

1/4 teaspoon salt

125ml of almond milk

1 egg

125g of fresh blueberries

1 tablespoon melted coconut oil

Preparation

Preheat the oven to 180°C. In a bowl, mix the flours, baking powder, bicarbonate of soda and salt. In another bowl, beat the eggs with the erythritol until the mixture becomes frothy. Add almond milk, coconut oil and mix well. Combine the two mixtures and gently incorporate the blueberries. Pour the mixture into the muffin molds lined with baking paper. Bake for 20-25 minutes, or until golden brown. Tips You can replace the blueberries with other berries or dried fruit. For a lactose-free version, use coconut or oat milk.

GREEK YOGURT WITH WALNUTS AND HONEY

Preparation time: 5 minutes

Servings: 2

Ingredients

300g of Greek yogurt

90g of coarsely chopped walnuts

2 tablespoon honey

Ground cinnamon to taste (optional)

Preparation

In a bowl, pour the Greek yogurt. Add chopped walnuts and honey. Stir gently to combine the ingredients. Sprinkle with a pinch of cinnamon, if desired. Tips You can customize the recipe by adding fresh fruit such as blueberries or strawberries. For a crunchy touch, you can lightly toast the nuts before adding them to the yogurt.

HERBAL OMELETTE WITH FETA AND PEPPERS

Preparation time: 10 minutes

Cooking time: 5 minutes

Servings: 1

Ingredients

2 eggs

1/2 red pepper

1/4 onion

30g of crumbled feta

A mix of fresh aromatic herbs

chopped (parsley, basil, oregano)

Salt and pepper to taste

Extra virgin olive oil

Preparation

Work the eggs in a bowl with a fork, adding salt and pepper. Finely chop the pepper and onion. In a non-stick pan, heat a drizzle of oil and fry the pepper and onion until tender. Add the beaten eggs to the pan and cook over medium heat, stirring gently with a spatula until the omelet is cooked. Crumble the feta and herbs over the omelette and serve immediately. Tips You can use other vegetables to taste, such as spinach or mushrooms. For a spicy twist, add chopped fresh chili pepper.

COCONUT FLOUR PANCAKES WITH MAPLE SYRUP

Preparation time: 15 minutes

Cooking time: 10 minutes

Servings: 4

Ingredients

100g of coconut flour

2 eggs

1 ripe banana

1/2 teaspoon baking powder

1 pinch of salt

Coconut milk to taste to get

a thick batter

Coconut oil to grease the pan

Maple syrup to taste for serving

Preparation

In a bowl, mash the banana with a fork. Add the eggs, coconut flour, baking powder and salt. Mix well. Gradually add the coconut milk until you obtain a thick and creamy batter. Heat a non-stick pan greased with coconut oil. Pour a ladle of batter for each pancake and cook for 2-3 minutes per side, or until golden brown. Serve hot with maple syrup. Tips You can add dried fruit or seeds to the batter for a crunchy touch. Serve pancakes with fresh fruit or sugar-free jam.

PARFAIT OF GREEK YOGURT GRANOLA AND STRAWBERRIES

Preparation time: 5 minutes

Servings: 2

Ingredients

300g of Greek yogurt

90g of granola

150g of fresh strawberries

Preparation

In a glass or cup, pour a layer of Greek yogurt. Add a layer of granola. Add a layer of chopped strawberries. Repeat the layers until you run out of ingredients. If desired, top with a drizzle of honey. Tips You can customize the parfait with other berries or fresh fruit to your liking. For a higher protein version, you can add chia or flax seeds to the yogurt.

RECIPES APPETIZERS

WHOLEMEAL BREAD BRUSCHETTA WITH CHERRY TOMATOES AND BASIL

Preparation time: 15 minutes

Cooking time: 5 minutes

(for grilling bread)

Doses: 4 people

Ingredients:

1 wholemeal baguette

250g cherry tomatoes

1 clove of garlic

Fresh basil to taste

Extra virgin olive oil to taste

Salt and pepper to taste

Preparation:

Preheat the oven grill. Cut the baguette into slices approximately 1 cm thick. Wash the cherry tomatoes and cut them in half. Rub the bread slices with garlic. Arrange the bread slices on a baking tray and grill until golden brown. In a bowl, combine the cherry tomatoes, chopped basil, oil, salt and pepper. Distribute the dressing over the hot bruschetta and serve.

GRILLED COURGETTE ROLL WITH RICOTTA AND WALNUTS

Preparation time: 20 minutes

Cooking time: 15 minutes

Doses: 4 people

Ingredients:

2 courgettes

250g ricotta

50g chopped walnuts

Fresh basil to taste

Salt and pepper to taste

Extra virgin olive oil to taste

Preparation:

Wash the courgettes and cut them into longitudinal slices. Grill the courgette slices until soft. In a bowl, mix the ricotta with the chopped walnuts, chopped basil, salt and pepper. Spread the ricotta mixture over each slice of grilled courgette. Roll up the courgettes and secure them with a toothpick. Arrange the rolls on a serving plate and drizzle with a drizzle of oil.

BOILED EGGS WITH LIGHT MAYONNAISE

Preparation Times: About 5 minutes

Cooking Times: 10-12 minutes for eggs

Doses Ingredients for 4 People:

8 hard boiled eggs

4 tablespoons light mayonnaise

Salt and black pepper to taste

Sweet paprika

(optional, for garnish)

Preparation:

Place the eggs in a saucepan and cover them with cold water. Bring the water to a boil, then reduce the heat and let the eggs cook for 10 to 12 minutes. Drain them and cool them under cold running water, then peel them. Cut the hard-boiled eggs in half lengthwise. Gently remove the egg yolks and place them in a bowl. Crush the egg yolks with a fork and mix with the light mayonnaise, salt and black pepper until you obtain a smooth cream. Fill the egg halves with the prepared yolk cream. Garnish with a sprinkle of sweet paprika (optional). Serve hard-boiled eggs with light mayonnaise as an appetizer or snack.

CURRY CHICKEN SKEWERS WITH YOGURT SAUCE

Preparation Times: About 20 minutes

Cooking Times: 10-15 minutes

Doses Ingredients for 4 People:

500g chicken breast, cut into cubes

2 tablespoons Greek yogurt

1 tablespoon curry powder

Juice of 1 lemon

Salt and black pepper to taste

Wood for skewers

(previously soaked in water)

Yogurt sauce

(see preparation below)

Preparation:

In a bowl, mix the Greek yogurt, curry powder, lemon juice, salt and pepper. Add the chicken cubes to the yogurt marinade and let them marinate in the refrigerator for at least 15-20 minutes. Thread the marinated chicken cubes onto the skewer sticks. Cook the chicken skewers on a grill or in a nonstick skillet until golden brown and fully cooked, about 10 to 15 minutes. Make the yogurt sauce by mixing Greek yogurt, a little curry powder and lemon juice. Serve the chicken skewers hot with the yogurt sauce as a dip.

AUBERGINES ROLLATINI WITH RICOTTA AND SPINACH

Preparation Times: About 30 minutes

Cooking Times: 25-30 minutes

Doses Ingredients for 4 People:

2 medium aubergines

250 g of fresh spinach

250 g of ricotta

1 cup tomato sauce

1 cup grated mozzarella cheese

2 tablespoons of olive oil

Salt and black pepper to taste

Fresh basil for garnish

Preparation:

Preheat the oven to 180°C (350°F). Cut the aubergines into long, thin slices. Heat a pan with olive oil and cook the aubergine slices until soft and lightly browned on both sides. Drain them on absorbent paper to remove excess oil. Meanwhile, in a separate pan, cook the spinach until wilted. Drain them and squeeze them to remove excess water. In a bowl, mix the ricotta and cooked spinach. Add salt and pepper to taste. Take a slice of eggplant, add a spoonful of the spinach-ricotta mixture, then roll up the eggplant. Arrange the aubergine rollatini in a baking pan, cover them with tomato sauce and grated mozzarella. Bake in the preheated oven for about 25-30 minutes or until the cheese is golden and melted. Garnish with fresh basil before serving.

TURKEY MEATBALLS WITH BASIL

Preparation Times: About 20 minutes

Cooking Times: 15-20 minutes

Doses Ingredients for 4 People:

500 g of minced turkey meat

1/2 cup breadcrumbs

(preferably whole)

1/4 cup grated Parmesan

1/4 cup chopped fresh basil

1 egg

2 cloves of garlic minced

Salt and black pepper to taste

2 tablespoons olive oil for cooking

Preparation:

In a bowl, mix the ground turkey, breadcrumbs, Parmesan cheese, fresh basil, egg, minced garlic, salt and pepper. Mix well until you obtain a homogeneous mixture. Form the mixture into small meatballs. Heat the olive oil in a nonstick skillet over medium heat. Cook turkey meatballs in skillet until golden brown and fully cooked, turning occasionally. It will take about 15-20 minutes. Drain the meatballs on absorbent paper to remove excess oil. Serve the turkey meatballs with basil as an appetizer or main course, as desired.

SMOKED SALMON WITH CREAM CHEESE AND CUCUMBER

Preparation Times: About 15 minutes

Cooking Times: No cooking

Doses Ingredients for 4 People:

200 g of smoked salmon (slices or steaks)

150 g of cream cheese

with reduced fat content

1 cucumber, thinly sliced

2 tablespoons finely chopped red onion

Juice of 1 lemon

Salt and black pepper to taste

Fresh dill for garnish (optional)

Preparation:

In a bowl, mix the cream cheese with the chopped red onion, lemon juice, salt and black pepper until smooth. Spread the smoked salmon slices or steaks on a serving plate. Spread the cream cheese over the surface of the salmon. Layer the thin cucumber slices on top of the cream cheese. Garnish with fresh dill (optional). Fold the smoked salmon on itself or leave it open, as desired. Serve smoked salmon with cream cheese and cucumber as an appetizer or snack.

AVOCADO STUFFED WITH TUNA AND BLACK OLIVES

Preparation Times: About 15 minutes

Cooking Times: No cooking

Doses Ingredients for 4 People:

2 ripe avocados, halved and pitted, 150g canned tuna, drained

1/4 cup pitted black olives, chopped

2 tablespoons finely chopped red onion

Juice of 1 lime, Salt and black pepper to taste

Preparation:

In a bowl, combine the drained tuna, chopped black olives, chopped red onion, lime juice, salt and black pepper. Fill the cavities of the avocados with the tuna and black olive mixture. Garnish with fresh parsley (optional). Serve stuffed avocados with tuna and black olives as an appetizer or snack.

MELON WRAPPED IN RAW HAM

Preparation Times: About 10 minutes

Cooking Times: No cooking

Doses Ingredients for 4 People:

1 ripe melon

8 slices of raw ham

Fresh mint leaves for

garnish (optional)

Preparation:

Cut the melon in half, remove the seeds and peel, then cut into thin slices or wedges, as desired. Wrap each slice or wedge of melon with a slice of cured ham. If desired, garnish with fresh mint leaves for a touch of freshness. Serve the melon wrapped in raw ham as an appetizer or snack.

TUNA TARTARE WITH AVOCADO

Preparation Times: About 20 minutes (refrigeration time included)

Cooking Times: No cooking

Doses Ingredients for 4 People:

300 g of fresh tuna, cut into small cubes

2 ripe avocados, cut into cubes

1/4 red onion, finely chopped

Juice of 1 lime

2 tablespoons extra virgin olive oil

Salt and black pepper to taste

Chopped fresh chili pepper (optional)

Fresh coriander leaves

for garnish (optional)

Preparation:

In a bowl, mix the diced tuna with the avocado, chopped red onion, lime juice, olive oil, salt and black pepper. Add chopped fresh chili pepper if you want a touch of heat. Cover the bowl and place it in the refrigerator for about 15-20 minutes to let the flavors blend. When ready to serve, garnish the tuna tartare with fresh coriander leaves, if desired. Serve tuna tartare with avocado as a starter or light main course.

GRILLED COURGETTES WITH DRIED TOMATO PESTO

Preparation Times: About 15 minutes

Cooking Times: 10-15 minutes

(for grilling the courgettes)

Doses Ingredients for 4 People:

4 medium courgettes

1/4 cup dried tomatoes in oil

2 tablespoons chopped walnuts

2 tablespoons grated Parmesan

2 tablespoons extra virgin olive oil

Juice of 1/2 lemon

Salt and black pepper to taste

Fresh basil leaves

for garnish (optional)

Preparation:

Preheat grill to medium-high heat. Cut the courgettes into long slices, brush them with a little olive oil and grill them until tender and lightly browned. Meanwhile, in a food processor, blend the dried tomatoes in oil, chopped walnuts, grated Parmesan cheese, lemon juice, olive oil, salt and black pepper until creamy. Arrange the grilled courgettes on a serving platter. Pour the sun-dried tomato pesto over the courgettes. Garnish with fresh basil leaves (optional). Serve the grilled zucchini with sun-dried tomato pesto as an appetizer or side dish.

BAKED AUBERGINES WITH TOMATO AND MOZZARELLA

Preparation Times: About 30 minutes

Cooking Times: 30-35 minutes

Doses Ingredients for 4 People:

2 medium aubergines

2 cups tomato sauce

200 g mozzarella, cut into cubes

1/4 cup grated Parmesan

2 tablespoons of olive oil

Salt and black pepper to taste

Fresh basil leaves for garnish

Preparation:

Preheat the oven to 180°C (350°F). Cut the aubergines into thin slices lengthwise. In a nonstick pan, sear the eggplant slices in olive oil until golden on both sides. In a baking pan, spread a layer of tomato sauce. Place a slice of eggplant on each spoonful of sauce, then cover them with mozzarella cubes. Repeat the process until you run out of ingredients, finishing with a final layer of sauce. Sprinkle grated Parmesan cheese on top. Bake in the preheated oven for about 30-35 minutes or until the cheese is golden and melted. Garnish with fresh basil leaves before serving.

CUCUMBERS STUFFED WITH SALMON AND CHEESE

Preparation Times: About 15 minutes

Cooking Times: No cooking

Doses Ingredients for 4 People:

4 cucumbers

200 g of smoked salmon,

cut into thin strips

100g light spreadable cheese

1 tablespoon chopped chives

Juice of 1/2 lemon

Salt and black pepper to taste

Fresh dill for garnish (optional)

Preparation:

Wash the cucumbers and peel them into strips, leaving some strips of peel for decoration. Cut each cucumber in half lengthwise and hollow them out with a teaspoon to remove the seeds. In a bowl, mix the light cream cheese with the chopped chives, lemon juice, salt and black pepper. Fill each cucumber half with the cheese mixture. Wrap each cucumber with strips of smoked salmon. Garnish with fresh dill (optional). Serve cucumbers stuffed with salmon and cheese as an appetizer or snack.

MUSHROOMS STUFFED WITH SAUSAGE AND CHEESE

Preparation Times: About 30 minutes

Cooking Times: 20-25 minutes

Doses Ingredients for 4 People:

12 large button mushrooms

200 g of crumbled sausage

1/2 cup ricotta cheese

1/4 cup grated Parmesan

2 tablespoons chopped fresh parsley

1 clove of garlic finely chopped

Salt and black pepper to taste

Breadcrumbs for garnish

Preparation:

Wash the mushrooms and remove the stems. In a pan, cook the crumbled sausage until well cooked, then drain to remove excess oil. In a bowl, mix the cooked sausage with the ricotta, grated Parmigiano Reggiano cheese, chopped fresh parsley, minced garlic, salt and black pepper. Fill the mushrooms with the sausage and cheese mixture. Sprinkle the stuffed mushrooms with a light amount of breadcrumbs. Place the stuffed mushrooms on a lightly greased baking tray. Bake in a preheated oven at 180°C (350°F) for approximately 20-25 minutes or until the mushrooms are tender and the breadcrumbs are golden. Serve the mushrooms stuffed with sausage and cheese as an appetizer or side dish.

MARINATED OLIVES WITH GARLIC AND ROSEMARY

Preparation Times: About 10 minutes

Cooking Times: No cooking

Doses Ingredients for 4 People:

2 cups green or black olives (stoneless)

2 cloves garlic, thinly sliced

2 sprigs of fresh rosemary

1/4 cup extra virgin olive oil

Grated lemon zest (optional)

Black pepper to taste

Preparation:

In a bowl, mix the olives with thinly sliced garlic, fresh rosemary sprigs and grated lemon zest (if you want a touch of freshness). Pour the extra virgin olive oil over the olives and mix well to coat them evenly. Add black pepper to taste for a touch of spiciness. Cover the bowl and let marinate in the refrigerator for at least 30 minutes or longer to develop the flavors. Before serving, remove the rosemary sprigs. Serve the marinated olives as an appetizer or snack.

COURGETTE FRITTERS WITH AROMATIC HERBS

Preparation Times: About 20 minutes

Cooking Times: 10-15 minutes

Doses Ingredients for 4 People:

2 medium courgettes

2 eggs

1/4 cup almond flour (or other
low carb flour)

2 tablespoons grated Parmesan

2 tablespoons chopped fresh herbs
(e.g. parsley, basil, chives)

Salt and black pepper to taste

Olive oil for cooking

Preparation:

Grate the courgettes and squeeze them to remove excess water. In a bowl, beat the eggs and then add the grated courgettes, almond flour, grated Parmigiano Reggiano cheese and chopped fresh aromatic herbs. Mix well until you obtain a homogeneous mixture. Heat a non-stick pan with a little olive oil over medium heat. Pour a heaping tablespoon of the zucchini mixture into the pan to form each pancake. Cook the courgette fritters for about 3-4 minutes per side, or until golden brown and cooked through. Drain them on absorbent paper to remove excess oil. Serve the zucchini fritters with herbs as an appetizer or side dish.

GRILLED PRAWN SKEWERS

Preparation Times: About 20 minutes (marinating time included)

Cooking Times: 5-7 minutes

Doses Ingredients for 4 People:

500 g large prawns, peeled and cleaned

Juice of 1 lemon

2 tablespoons of olive oil

2 cloves of garlic finely chopped

1 teaspoon sweet paprika

Salt and black pepper to taste

Fresh rosemary sprigs

for the skewers (optional)

Preparation:

In a bowl, mix the lemon juice, olive oil, minced garlic, sweet paprika, salt and black pepper to create the marinade. Add the shrimp to the marinade and mix well to coat them evenly. Leave to marinate in the refrigerator for at least 15-20 minutes. Preheat grill to medium-high heat. Thread the marinated prawns into the rosemary sprigs or onto wooden skewers previously soaked in water. Grill the prawn skewers for about 2-3 minutes per side, or until pink and cooked through. Serve the grilled shrimp skewers as an appetizer or main course.

GUACAMOLE WITH ZUCCHINI CHIPS

Preparation Times: About 15 minutes

Cooking Times: 10-12 minutes

Doses Ingredients for 4 People:

4 medium courgettes

2 ripe avocados

Juice of 2 lemons

1 tomato, peeled and chopped

1/4 red onion, finely chopped

2 cloves of garlic finely chopped

1/4 cup chopped fresh cilantro

Salt and black pepper to taste

Chopped fresh chili pepper (optional)

Preparation:

Preheat the oven to 180°C (350°F). Cut the courgettes into thin slices. Place the courgette slices on a baking tray, brush them with a little olive oil, then cook in the preheated oven for about 10-12 minutes or until crispy. Turn the slices over halfway through cooking. While the courgettes are cooking, prepare the guacamole. In a bowl, mash the avocados with a fork and mix with the lemon juice, chopped tomato, red onion, chopped garlic, fresh cilantro, salt and black pepper. Add chopped fresh chili pepper if you want a spicy kick. Once ready, serve the crispy zucchini chips with guacamole as an appetizer or snack.

BOILED QUAIL EGGS WITH SALT AND PEPPER

Preparation Times: About 5 minutes

Cooking Times: 3-4 minutes

Doses Ingredients for 4 People:

16 quail eggs

Salt and black pepper to taste

Flaked sea salt for presentation (optional)

Preparation:

In a saucepan, bring some water to the boil and add a pinch of salt. Gently lower the quail eggs into the boiling water with a slotted spoon. Cook the quail eggs for 3-4 minutes to obtain hard-boiled eggs, then drain them and immerse them in cold water to stop the cooking. Once cooled, peel the quail eggs. Cut each quail egg in half, sprinkle with a pinch of salt and black pepper. If you want an elegant presentation, you can sprinkle some flaked sea salt on top of the eggs. Serve hard-boiled quail eggs as an appetizer or snack.

CHEESE BALLS WITH VALNUTS

Preparation Times: About 15 minutes

Cooking Times: No cooking

Doses Ingredients for 4 People:

200 g of cream cheese

with reduced fat content

1/2 cup chopped walnuts

2 tablespoons of chives

finely chopped

Black pepper to taste

Preparation:

In a bowl, mix the reduced-fat cream cheese with chopped walnuts, finely chopped chives and a generous grind of black pepper. Mix well until you obtain a homogeneous mixture. Take small portions of the mixture and form small balls of cheese with your hands. Arrange the cheese balls on a serving plate. If desired, additionally sprinkle with black pepper or chives to decorate. Serve the cheese balls with nuts as an appetizer or snack.

BRUSCHETTA WITH TOMATO AND BASIL ON WHOLEMEAL BREAD

Preparation Times: 15 minutes

Doses Ingredients for 4 People:

4 slices of wholemeal bread

(about 1cm thick)

2 ripe tomatoes, 1-2 cloves of garlic

Fresh basil leaves

Extra virgin olive oil

Salt and black pepper to taste

Preparation

Make the Bread: Preheat the oven broiler or use a broiler to toast the wholemeal bread until golden brown on both sides.

You can also toast the bread in a non-stick pan with a drizzle of olive oil. Prepare the Tomatoes: Wash the tomatoes and cut them into small cubes. Remove the seeds to prevent the bruschetta from becoming too moist. Flavor Olive Oil: In a small bowl, mix 2-3 tablespoons extra virgin olive oil with a finely chopped clove of garlic. Let the garlic infuse the oil for a more intense flavor. Assemble the Bruschettas: Lightly rub another clove of garlic on the surface of the toasted bread slices. This will add a hint of garlic flavor to the bread. Distribute the tomato cubes evenly on the toasted bread slices. Add a few fresh basil leaves on top of the tomatoes. Season with salt and pepper to taste. Drizzle the flavored olive oil over the entire bruschetta. Serve and Enjoy: Arrange the bruschetta on a serving plate. Serve immediately as a moderate carb appetizer.

CROSTINI WITH HUMMUS AND DRIED TOMATOES

Preparation Times: Approximately 10-15 minutes

ìCooking Times: No cooking

Doses Ingredients for 4 People:

1 wholemeal baguette or 4-6 slices of wholemeal bread

1 cup hummus

1/2 cup dried tomatoes in oil,

drained and cut into strips

Fresh basil leaves for garnish (optional)

Extra virgin olive oil

Salt and black pepper to taste

Preparation:

Preheat the oven broiler or use a broiler to toast the wholemeal bread until golden brown on both sides. Spread a generous amount of hummus on each crostini. Place the dried tomato strips on top of the hummus. Add salt and pepper to taste. If desired, garnish with fresh basil leaves. Arrange the croutons on a serving plate. Serve them as an appetizer or snack.

CHICKEN MEATBALLS

WITH BBQ SAUCE

Preparation Times: Approximately 15-20 minutes

Cooking Times: Approximately 10-15 minutes

Doses Ingredients for 4 People:

500 g of minced chicken meat

1/2 onion, finely chopped

1 clove garlic, finely chopped

1 egg

1/4 cup breadcrumbs or flour

of almonds (to make meatballs low carb)

2 tablespoons chopped fresh parsley

Salt and black pepper to taste

Olive oil for cooking

Preparation:

In a bowl, mix the ground chicken, chopped onion, minced garlic, egg, breadcrumbs or almond flour, chopped fresh parsley, salt and black pepper. Mix well until you obtain a homogeneous mixture. Take small portions of the mixture and shape into round, compact meatballs. In a nonstick skillet, heat some olive oil over medium heat. Cook meatballs until golden brown and fully cooked, turning occasionally. It will take about 10-15 minutes. Serve and Enjoy: Serve the chicken meatballs with BBQ sauce as an appetizer or main course.

POTATO SALAD WITH GREEK YOGURT AND MUSTARD

Preparation Times: Approximately 15-20 minutes

Cooking Times: Approximately 15-20 minutes

Doses Ingredients for 4 People:

500 g yellow-fleshed potatoes,

peeled and cut into cubes

1/2 cup Greek yogurt

1 tablespoon Dijon mustard

2 tablespoons light mayonnaise

2 tablespoons finely chopped red onion

2 tablespoons finely chopped pickled gherkins

Salt and black pepper to taste

Chopped fresh parsley for garnish (optional)

Preparation:

Cook the potato cubes in lightly salted water until they become tender, then drain and leave to cool. In a large bowl, combine Greek yogurt, Dijon mustard, mayonnaise, chopped red onion, chopped gherkins, salt, and black pepper. Add the cooled potatoes to the seasoning mix and toss gently until the potatoes are evenly coated. Garnish with chopped fresh parsley, if desired. Cover the salad and let it cool in the refrigerator for at least an hour before serving. Serve potato salad as a side dish or light main course.

CHICKEN WRAPS WITH GRILLED VEGETABLES

Preparation Times: Approximately 20-25 minutes

Cooking Times: Approximately 10-15 minutes

Doses Ingredients for 4 People:

For the Marinated Chicken:

500 g chicken breast cut into strips

2 tablespoons of olive oil

2 tablespoons lemon juice

1 clove of garlic finely chopped

1 teaspoon sweet paprika

Salt and black pepper to taste

For the grilled vegetables:

A selection of vegetables such as peppers,

courgettes and onions, cut into strips

Olive oil for marinating

Salt and black pepper to taste

For Seasoning and Assembling:

4 wholemeal tortillas or wraps

Lettuce leaves

Tzatziki sauce or sauce based

of Greek yogurt (optional)

Preparation:

For the Marinated Chicken: In a bowl, combine the olive oil, lemon juice, minced garlic, sweet paprika, salt and black pepper. Add the chicken breast strips and let them marinate for at least 15-20 minutes. For the Grilled Vegetables: Marinate the vegetable strips with olive oil, salt and pepper. Grill vegetables until tender and lightly smoky. For Seasoning and Assembling:

Cook the marinated chicken in a skillet or on a grill until cooked through and golden brown. Reheat whole-wheat tortillas. For each tortilla, top with a few lettuce leaves, grilled chicken, grilled vegetables, and a generous dollop of tzatziki sauce or other Greek yogurt-based dip (if desired). Roll the tortilla to create the wrap. Serve the chicken wraps with grilled vegetables as a main course or snack.

SWEET POTATO NACHOS WITH AVOCADO SAUCE

Preparation Times: Approximately 15-20 minutes

Cooking Times: Approximately 20-25 minutes

Doses Ingredients for 4 People:

For the Sweet Potato Nachos:

2 large sweet potatoes, peeled and thinly sliced

2 tablespoons of olive oil

Salt, black pepper and smoked paprika to taste

For the Avocado Sauce:

2 ripe avocados, peeled and pitted

Juice of 1 lemon

1 clove of garlic finely chopped

1/4 red onion finely chopped

Salt and black pepper to taste

Fresh coriander leaves for garnish

Preparation:

For the Sweet Potato Nachos: Preheat the oven to 200°C. In a bowl, toss the sweet potato slices with the olive oil, salt, black pepper, and smoked paprika until well coated. Spread the potato slices on a baking tray lined with baking paper. Bake for 20-25 minutes or until sweet potatoes are crispy. For the Avocado Salsa: In a bowl, mash the avocados with a fork.

Add lemon juice, minced garlic, chopped red onion, fresh chili pepper (if you want a spicy kick), salt and black pepper. Mix well until you get a creamy sauce. Assembly: Arrange the sweet potato nachos on a serving platter. Serve with avocado salsa over nachos. Garnish with fresh coriander leaves. Serve as an appetizer or snack.

QUINOA SALAD WITH ROASTED VEGETABLES

Preparation Times: Approximately 20-25 minutes

Cooking Times: Approximately 25-30 minutes

Doses Ingredients for 4 People:

For the Quinoa Salad:

1 cup quinoa

2 cups water or vegetable broth

2 cups mixed vegetables (such as peppers, courgettes, tomatoes, onions), cut into cubes

2 tablespoons of olive oil

Salt and black pepper to taste

For the seasoning:

3 tablespoons of olive oil

Juice of 1 lemon

1 teaspoon honey or maple syrup

Salt and black pepper to taste

Fresh parsley leaves for garnish

Preparation:

For the Quinoa Salad: Rinse the quinoa under cold running water. In a saucepan, bring 2 cups water or vegetable broth to a boil. Add the quinoa, cover and reduce the heat to low. Cook for 15-20 minutes or until the quinoa has absorbed the liquid and is cooked. While the quinoa cooks, heat 2 tablespoons olive oil in a skillet and cook the diced vegetables until tender and lightly roasted. When the quinoa is ready, fluff it with a fork and let it cool.

For the Dressing: In a bowl, combine the olive oil, lemon juice, honey or maple syrup, salt and black pepper. Assembly: In a large bowl, mix the cooked and cooled quinoa with the roasted vegetables. Pour the dressing over the salad and mix well. Garnish with fresh parsley leaves. Serve the quinoa salad as a main course or side dish.

SMOKED SALMON ROLLS WITH CHEESE

Preparation Times: Approximately 15-20 minutes

Cooking Times: No cooking

Doses Ingredients for 4 People:

200 g smoked salmon (thinly sliced)

200 g cream cheese (you can use spreadable cheese of your choice)

Fresh chives (for garnish, optional)

Ground black pepper to taste

Lemon (for garnish, optional)

Preparation:

Lay out the smoked salmon slices on a clean work surface. Spread cream cheese on each salmon slice. Add a pinch of ground black pepper to each slice. If you like, you can add some chopped fresh chives on top of the cheese. Gently roll the salmon with the cheese inside, forming rolls. Cut the rolls in half or into bite-sized pieces, if desired. If desired, garnish with lemon slices.

CHICKPEA MEATBALLS WITH YOGURT SAUCE

Preparation Times: Approximately 15-20 minutes

Cooking Times: Approximately 15-20 minutes

Doses Ingredients for 4 People:

For the chickpea meatballs:

2 cans chickpeas, drained and rinsed

1/2 red onion, finely chopped

2 cloves garlic, finely chopped

2 tablespoons chopped fresh parsley

1 teaspoon cumin powder

1 teaspoon sweet paprika

Salt and black pepper to taste

2 tablespoons chickpea flour (or other flour

to your liking) for the dough

Olive oil for cooking

For the Yogurt Sauce:

1 cup Greek yogurt

Juice of 1/2 lemon

1 teaspoon honey or maple syrup

Salt and black pepper to taste

Chopped fresh parsley for garnish

Preparation:

For the Chickpea Meatballs: In a food processor, blend the drained chickpeas, chopped red onion, chopped garlic, chopped fresh parsley, powdered cumin, sweet paprika, salt and black pepper until smooth. a homogeneous compound. Add the chickpea flour and mix until the mixture becomes thick enough to form meatballs.

Shape meatballs with your hands and place them on a plate. Heat some olive oil in a pan and cook the meatballs until golden brown on both sides. For the Yogurt Sauce: In a bowl, combine the Greek yogurt, lemon juice, honey or maple syrup, salt and black pepper. Serve the chickpea meatballs with the yogurt sauce and garnish with chopped fresh parsley.

EGG SALAD WITH

BACON AND SPINACH

Preparation Times: Approximately 15-20 minutes

Cooking Times: Approximately 10-15 minutes

6 hard-boiled eggs, peeled and cut in half

4 cups fresh spinach, washed and dried

150g crispy bacon, cut into cubes

1/2 red onion, finely chopped

1/4 cup crumbled feta cheese

2 tablespoons toasted sunflower seeds

(optional for crunchiness)

Extra virgin olive oil

Salt and black pepper to taste

Vinaigrette to your liking (optional)

Preparation:

In a skillet, cook bacon over medium-high heat until crisp. Drain the excess oil and let it cool on absorbent paper. In a large bowl, arrange the fresh spinach. Place the hard-boiled eggs cut in half on top of the spinach. Spread the crispy bacon and chopped red onion over the eggs. Add crumbled feta cheese and toasted sunflower seeds (if using). Season with a drizzle of extra virgin olive oil, salt and black pepper to taste. You can also add a vinaigrette of your choice for an extra touch of flavor.

SAVORY PIE WITH BROCCOLI AND CHEESE

Preparation Times: Approximately 20-25 minutes

Cooking Times: Approximately 30-35 minutes

Doses Ingredients for 4 People:

1 rectangular puff pastry (about 230 g)

2 cups fresh broccoli, chopped and blanched

1 cup shredded cheddar cheese

4 eggs

1/2 cup milk

1 clove of garlic finely chopped

Salt and black pepper to taste

Nutmeg to taste

Preparation:

Preheat the oven to 180°C and line a rectangular baking tray with baking paper. Roll out the puff pastry in the pan, making sure to completely cover the bottom and edges. In a bowl, beat the eggs with the milk, minced garlic, grated cheddar cheese, salt, black pepper and a grating of nutmeg. Spread the blanched broccoli over the puff pastry. Pour the egg and cheese mixture over the broccoli. Bake in the preheated oven for about 30-35 minutes or until the cake is golden brown and the inside is set. Let cool slightly before cutting the cake into slices and serving.

CHICKEN SANDWICHES WITH PESTO AND LETTUCE

Preparation Times: Approximately 15-20 minutes

Cooking Times: Approximately 10-15 minutes

Doses Ingredients for 4 People:

4 wholemeal rolls or sesame rolls

4 skinless, boneless chicken breasts

4 tablespoons pesto (you can use pesto purchased or prepare it at home)

Lettuce leaves

Sliced tomatoes (optional)

Cheese of your choice (optional)

Salt and black pepper to taste

Olive oil for cooking

Preparation:

Heat some olive oil in a pan or on a grill. Season the chicken breasts with salt and black pepper. Cook the chicken until fully cooked and browned on both sides, usually 5-7 minutes per side, depending on the thickness of the chicken breast. During the last few minutes of cooking, spread pesto on both sides of the chicken for flavor. Cut the buns in half and toast lightly if desired. Assemble the sandwiches with a lettuce leaf, a slice of tomato (if desired), chicken breast with pesto and cheese (if using). Serve chicken sandwiches as hot sandwiches for a delicious lunch or snack.

TURKEY SKEWERS WITH TZATZIKI SAUCE

Preparation Times: Approximately 20-25 minutes

Cooking Times: Approximately 10-15 minutes

Doses Ingredients for 4 People:

For the Turkey Skewers:

500 g turkey breast cut into cubes

1 lemon, juice and zest

2 tablespoons of olive oil

2 teaspoons dried oregano

Salt and black pepper to taste

Wooden skewer sticks (soaked

in water to prevent them from burning)

For the Tzatziki Sauce:

1 cup Greek yogurt

1 cucumber, peeled, seeded and grated

2 cloves of garlic finely chopped

Juice of 1/2 lemon

2 tablespoons extra virgin olive oil

1 tablespoon chopped fresh mint (optional)

Salt and black pepper to taste

Preparation:

For the Turkey Skewers: In a bowl, combine the lemon juice and zest, olive oil, dried oregano, salt and black pepper. Thread the turkey breast cubes onto the previously soaked skewer sticks. Brush the turkey cubes with the lemon-oregano marinade.

Cook the skewers on a hot grill or in a nonstick skillet until the turkey is fully cooked, usually 10 to 15 minutes. For the Tzatziki Sauce: In a bowl, combine Greek yogurt, grated cucumber, minced garlic, lemon juice, olive oil, fresh mint (if desired), salt, and black pepper . Let it rest in the refrigerator for at least 30 minutes before serving. Serve turkey skewers with tzatziki sauce as a main dish or snack.

CROSTINI WITH PORCINI MUSHROOMS AND CHEESE

Preparation Times: Approximately 20-25 minutes

Cooking Times: Approximately 10-15 minutes

Doses Ingredients for 4 People:

8 slices of baguette or ciabatta bread

200 g of fresh, cleaned porcini mushrooms and

sliced thinly (you can also use

soaked dried porcini mushrooms)

200 g cream cheese (you can

use your favorite spreadable cheese)

2 cloves garlic, finely chopped

Chopped fresh parsley for garnish

Extra virgin olive oil

Salt and black pepper to taste

Preparation:

Preheat the oven to 180°C. Place the bread slices on a baking tray and brush a little olive oil on both sides. Toast the bread slices in the oven until golden, about 5-7 minutes per side. Keep an eye on this as roasting time may vary. While the bread is toasting, heat some olive oil in a pan. Add the chopped garlic cloves and sliced porcini mushrooms and cook until the mushrooms are tender and golden. Add salt and black pepper to taste. Once toasted, spread the cream cheese on each slice of toast. Spread the sautéed porcini mushrooms on each crouton with cheese. Garnish with chopped fresh parsley. Serve the crostini as an appetizer or snack.

COUSCOUS SALAD WITH CUCUMBERS AND TOMATOES

Preparation Times: Approximately 15-20 minutes

Cooking Times: About 5 minutes

Doses Ingredients for 4 People:

1 cup couscous

1 cup boiling water

2 tablespoons extra virgin olive oil

Juice of 1 lemon

2 cucumbers, peeled and cut into cubes

2 ripe tomatoes, cut into cubes

1/2 red onion, finely chopped

Chopped fresh parsley to taste

Salt and black pepper to taste

Preparation:

In a bowl, pour the couscous. Pour the boiling water over the couscous, cover the bowl with a lid or a sheet of cling film and let it rest for about 5 minutes. After resting, fluff the couscous with a fork to make it light and airy. Add the olive oil and lemon juice to the couscous and mix well. Add the cucumbers, tomatoes, red onion, fresh parsley and season with salt and black pepper to taste. Mix everything carefully until you have a well-combined couscous salad. Serve the salad as a side or light main course.

AUBERGINES BRUSCHETTE WITH PARMESAN

Preparation Times: Approximately 30-35 minutes

Cooking Times: Approximately 20-25 minutes

Doses Ingredients for 4 People:

For the Bruschetta:

1 baguette or rustic bread

2 medium aubergines, thinly sliced

Extra virgin olive oil

Salt and black pepper to taste

2 cups diced peeled tomatoes (you can use fresh or canned tomatoes)

200 g fresh mozzarella, cut into cubes

1/2 cup grated Parmesan

Fresh basil for garnish

Preparation:

Preheat the oven to 200°C. Brush the eggplant slices with olive oil, salt and black pepper, then grill or broil the eggplant until tender and lightly browned. Cut the bread into thick slices and toast it lightly. In a skillet, heat the diced peeled tomatoes over medium-low heat and add salt and pepper to taste. Cook until the tomatoes thicken slightly. Assemble the bruschetta: place a layer of grilled aubergines on the toasted bread, then add the peeled tomatoes, diced mozzarella and grated Parmesan. Bake the bruschetta in the preheated oven for 5-7 minutes or until the cheese is melted and golden. Garnish with fresh basil leaves and serve the bruschetta as an appetizer or main course.

BEAN SALAD WITH TUNA AND RED ONION

Preparation Times: Approximately 15-20 minutes

Cooking Times: No cooking

Doses Ingredients for 4 People:

2 cans of cannellini beans or kidney beans

borlotti beans, drained and rinsed 2 cans of canned tuna, drained

1 red onion, thinly sliced

1 red pepper, cut into cubes

1/4 cup chopped fresh parsley

1/4 cup extra virgin olive oil

Juice of 1 lemon

Salt and black pepper to taste

Preparation:

In a large bowl, combine the drained cannellini beans, drained tuna, sliced red onion, diced red pepper and chopped fresh parsley. In a small bowl, prepare the vinaigrette by mixing the olive oil, lemon juice, salt, and black pepper to taste. Pour the vinaigrette over the bean and tuna salad and mix well until all the ingredients are well combined. Let the salad sit in the refrigerator for at least 30 minutes before serving to allow the flavors to blend. Serve the bean salad as a side dish or light main course.

QUINOA MEATBALLS WITH CHILLI SAUCE

Preparation Times: Approximately 30-35 minutes

Cooking Times: Approximately 15-20 minutes

Doses Ingredients for 4 People:

For the Meatballs:

1 cup quinoa

2 cups of water

1 egg

1/2 cup shredded cheese of your choice

(for example parmesan or pecorino)

2 tablespoons of breadcrumbs

2 cloves garlic, finely chopped

2 tablespoons chopped fresh parsley

Salt and black pepper to taste

Olive oil for cooking

For the Chilli Sauce:

1/2 cup Greek yogurt

1 fresh red chilli, finely chopped

Juice of 1 lime

Salt and black pepper to taste

Preparation:

Rinse the quinoa well under running water. In a saucepan, bring water to a boil, add quinoa and cook according to package instructions (usually about 15 minutes). Drain any excess water and let cool. In a large bowl, combine the cooked quinoa, egg, shredded cheese, breadcrumbs, minced garlic, chopped fresh parsley, salt and black pepper.

Mix until you obtain a homogeneous mixture. With wet hands, shape the quinoa mixture into meatballs. Heat some olive oil in a non-stick pan and cook the meatballs until golden brown on both sides. Meanwhile, make the chili sauce by mixing the Greek yogurt, crushed red chili pepper, lime juice, salt, and black pepper in a bowl. Serve the quinoa meatballs hot with the chili sauce as a condiment.

COURGETTE OMELETTE WITH GOAT'S CHEESE

Preparation Times: Approximately 20-25 minutes

Cooking Times: Approximately 10-15 minutes

Doses Ingredients for 4 People:

6 eggs

2 medium courgettes, cut into thin rounds

100g goat's cheese, crumbled

2 tablespoons extra virgin olive oil

1 red onion, finely chopped

Salt and black pepper to taste

Chopped fresh parsley for garnish (optional)

Preparation:

In a nonstick skillet, heat the olive oil over medium-high heat. Add the zucchini and chopped onion and cook until the zucchini is tender and lightly browned, about 5 to 7 minutes. Add salt and black pepper to taste. In a bowl, whisk the eggs and pour them over the zucchini and onion in the pan. Sprinkle the crumbled goat cheese over the top of the eggs. Cook over medium-low heat until the eggs are set and the cheese is melted, usually 10-15 minutes. Garnish with chopped fresh parsley, if desired. Serve zucchini omelette with goat cheese as a main course or appetizer.

HAM AND MELON ROLLS

Preparation Times: 15-20 minutes

Ingredients for 4 people:

1 ripe melon

200 g of raw ham

Fresh basil leaves

Ground black pepper

Preparation

Cut the melon in half, remove the seeds and use a spoon to create small balls or cubes of melon. You can also use a melon corer if you have one. Take a slice of cured ham and wrap it around each ball or cube of melon. Place the rolls on a serving plate. Take some fresh basil leaves and place them on top of the rolls. Add a grind of black pepper to the top of the rolls for a pop of flavor. Serve the ham and melon rolls as an appetizer. They are fresh, sweet and savory at the same time, perfect for stimulating the appetite.

RECIPES
FIRST DISHES

WHOLEMEAL RISOTTO WITH MUSHROOMS AND SPINACH

Preparation time: 20 minutes

Cooking time: 20-25 minutes

Doses: 4 people

Ingredients:

320g brown rice

1 liter vegetable broth

300g mixed mushrooms

200g fresh spinach

1 onion

2 cloves of garlic

50g butter

50g grated parmesan

Extra virgin olive oil

Salt and pepper to taste

Preparation:

Prepare the broth: Bring the vegetable broth to the boil and keep it warm. Sauteed: In a saucepan, melt the butter with the oil. Add the chopped onion and garlic and sauté. Toast the rice: Add the rice and toast it for a few minutes, stirring constantly, until it becomes transparent. Deglaze with a ladle of hot broth. Cooking: Continue cooking the risotto, adding the hot broth little at a time and stirring constantly. Mushrooms and spinach: In the meantime, clean the mushrooms and cut them into slices. Sauté them in a pan with a drizzle of oil until they are golden. Wash the spinach and blanch them for a few minutes. Completion: Halfway through cooking the risotto, add the sautéed mushrooms. Once cooked, stir in the risotto with the parmesan, spinach and ground pepper.

WHOLEMEAL PASTA WITH COURGETTES AND SMOKED SALMON

Preparation time: 15 minutes

Cooking time: 10 minutes

Doses: 4 people

Ingredients:

320g wholemeal pasta (fusilli, spaghetti or other form of your choice)

2 courgettes

200g smoked salmon

1 shallot

Extra virgin olive oil

Juice of half a lemon

Fresh mint (optional)

Salt and pepper to taste

Preparation:

Cook the pasta: Cook the pasta in plenty of salted water. Courgettes: In the meantime, wash the courgettes, cut them into julienne strips and sauté them in a pan with the chopped shallots and a drizzle of oil until they are tender. Seasoning: Crumble the smoked salmon and add it to the courgettes. Add lemon juice, salt, pepper and mix well. Service: Drain the pasta al dente and season it with the courgette and salmon sauce. If desired, add a few chopped fresh mint leaves.

ZUCCHINI SPAGHETTI WITH CHICKEN MEATBALLS

Preparation Times: 30-35 minutes

Cooking Times: 15-20 minutes

Doses Ingredients for 4 People:

For the Zucchini Spaghetti:

4 medium courgettes

Salt and black pepper to taste

For the Chicken Meatballs:

500 g of minced chicken meat

1/4 cup breadcrumbs

1 egg

2 tablespoons grated Parmesan

2 cloves garlic, minced

2 tablespoons chopped fresh parsley

Salt and black pepper to taste

Olive oil for cooking

Preparation:

Use a zucchini slicer or julienne cutter to create zucchini spaghetti. In a bowl, mix the ground chicken meat, breadcrumbs, egg, grated cheese, garlic, parsley, salt and pepper. Shape meatballs with your hands. Heat some olive oil in a non-stick pan and cook the chicken meatballs until golden and cooked through. While the meatballs are cooking, heat some olive oil in another pan and cook the zucchini spaghetti until tender but still crunchy. Serve the Zucchini Spaghetti with the Chicken Meatballs as desired.

SHRIMP AND AVOCADO SALAD WITH LIME SAUCE

Preparation Times: 20-25 minutes

Cooking Times: 5-7 minutes

Doses Ingredients for 4 People:

400 g of peeled and cleaned prawns

2 ripe avocados, cut into cubes

Juice of 2 limes

1/4 cup fresh cilantro, chopped

1 fresh red chilli, finely chopped

(optional for a spicy touch)

Salt and black pepper to taste

Extra virgin olive oil

Preparation:

If the prawns are not already cooked, cook them in a non-stick pan with a little olive oil until pink and opaque. In a bowl, combine cooked shrimp (cooled), diced avocados, lime juice, cilantro, red chili pepper (if using), salt, and pepper. Mix all the ingredients well and make sure the avocados are well coated in the lime sauce. Serve the Shrimp and Avocado Salad as desired.

EGG OMELETE WITH SPINACH AND CHEESE

Preparation Times: 15-20 minutes

Cooking Times: 10-15 minutes

Doses Ingredients for 4 People:

8 eggs

200 g of fresh spinach

1/2 cup grated cheese (e.g.

cheddar cheese or Swiss cheese)

Salt and black pepper to taste

Olive oil for cooking

Preparation:

In a nonstick skillet, heat some olive oil over medium heat. Add fresh spinach and cook until slightly wilted. In a bowl, beat the eggs, add the grated cheese, salt and pepper. Mix well. Pour the egg mixture over the spinach in the skillet. Cook the omelette over medium-low heat until it is set and the cheese is melted, usually 10-15 minutes. Serve the Egg Omelette with Spinach and Cheese as a main course.

ZUCCHINI SPAGHETTI WITH GARLIC BUTTER SAUCE

Preparation Times: 15-20 minutes

Cooking Times: 10-15 minutes

Doses Ingredients for 4 People:

4 medium courgettes

4 tablespoons butter

4 cloves garlic, finely chopped

Salt and black pepper to taste

Grated parmesan to taste (for garnish)

Chopped fresh parsley to taste (for garnish)

Preparation:

Use a zucchini slicer or julienne cutter to create zucchini spaghetti. In a skillet, melt the butter over medium-low heat. Add the minced garlic and cook until starting to brown. Add the zucchini noodles to the pan with the butter sauce and cook for 3-5 minutes or until tender but still crunchy. Add salt and pepper to taste. Serve Zucchini Spaghetti with Garlic Butter Sauce as a main course, garnished with grated Parmesan and chopped fresh parsley if desired.

BAKED SALMON ON A BED OF SPINACH

Preparation Times: 10-15 minutes

Cooking Times: 15-20 minutes

Doses Ingredients for 4 People:

4 salmon fillets (about 150 g each)

200 g of fresh spinach

Juice of 1 lemon

2 cloves garlic, finely chopped

Salt and black pepper to taste

Extra virgin olive oil

Lemon slices (for garnish)

Preparation:

Preheat the oven to 180°C. In a pan, heat some olive oil and add fresh spinach. Cook them until they wilt. Add the minced garlic and cook for a minute. Arrange the cooked spinach on a baking tray as a "bed" for the salmon. Place the salmon fillets on top of the spinach beds. Squeeze the lemon juice over the salmon and add salt and pepper to taste. Cover the pan with foil and bake for 15-20 minutes or until the salmon is cooked through and flakes easily with a fork. Garnish with lemon slices before serving.

CARPACCIO OF ZUCCHINI WITH DRIED TOMATOES AND CHEESE

Preparation Times: 10-15 minutes

Cooking Times: None (cold dish)

Doses Ingredients for 4 People:

2-3 medium courgettes

Dried tomatoes in oil, cut into strips

Cheese of your choice (e.g. parmesan, pecorino), grated or cut into flakes

Extra virgin olive oil

Lemon juice

Salt and black pepper to taste

Fresh basil leaves (for garnish)

Preparation:

Use a mandolin or potato peeler to slice the courgettes very thinly and arrange them in an even layer on a serving platter. Distribute the dried tomato strips over the courgettes. Add the grated or flaked cheese over the courgette and dried tomato carpaccio. Season with olive oil, lemon juice, salt and pepper to taste. Garnish with fresh basil leaves. Serve the Courgette Carpaccio with Dried Tomatoes and Cheese as an appetizer or side dish.

GHERKIN PAD THAI WITH GRILLED CHICKEN

Preparation Times: 20-25 minutes

Cooking Times: 10-15 minutes

Doses Ingredients for 4 People:

For the Gherkin Pad Thai:

4 spiral gherkins

2 grilled chicken breasts, cut into thin strips

2 eggs

1/4 cup soy sauce

2 tablespoons of brown sugar

Juice of 2 limes

2 cloves garlic, finely chopped

Chopped dry red chili pepper (to taste)

Olive oil for cooking

Preparation:

In a large pan, heat some olive oil and add the minced garlic. Cook until fragrant. Add the chicken to the grill and cook until cooked through and browned. Move the chicken to a plate and in the same pan, add the beaten eggs. Stir until thickened. Add the spiralized gherkins to the pan along with the eggs. Cook for a few minutes until tender but still crunchy. Add the soy sauce, brown sugar, lime juice, and dried red chili pepper (if using). Mix well. Add chicken to skillet and stir to combine all ingredients. Serve Gherkin Pad Thai with Grilled Chicken hot.

GRILLED AUBERGINES WITH TOMATO PESTO

Preparation Times: 15-20 minutes

Cooking Times: 10-15 minutes

Doses Ingredients for 4 People:

2 medium aubergines, cut into slices

Extra virgin olive oil

Salt and black pepper to taste

For the Tomato Pesto:

1 cup sun-dried tomatoes in oil, drained

2 cloves of garlic

1/4 cup fresh basil

1/4 cup grated Parmesan

Salt and black pepper to taste

Preparation:

Preheat a grill or grill plate. Brush the eggplant slices with olive oil, then grill them until tender and have classic grill streaks. Meanwhile, prepare the tomato pesto. In a blender, blend the sun-dried tomatoes, garlic, basil, grated cheese, salt and pepper until creamy. When the aubergines are ready, place them on a serving plate and sprinkle them with the tomato pesto. Serve the Grilled Eggplant with Tomato Pesto as an appetizer or side dish.

COURGETTE LASAGNE WITH RICOTTA AND MEAT SAUCE

Preparation Times: 30-40 minutes

Cooking Times: 30-35 minutes

Doses Ingredients for 4 People:

4 medium courgettes, cut into long slices

500 g minced meat (beef or pork)

1 onion, chopped, 2 cloves garlic, chopped

1 cup tomato sauce

1 cup cottage cheese

1/2 cup grated Parmesan

1/4 cup fresh basil, chopped

Salt and black pepper to taste

Extra virgin olive oil

Preparation:

Preheat the oven to 180°C. In a pan, heat some olive oil and add the chopped onion and garlic. Cook until golden brown. Add the ground beef and cook until well browned. Add the tomato sauce, salt and pepper. Cook for a few minutes. In a bowl, mix the ricotta, grated cheese and fresh basil. Add salt and pepper to taste. On a baking sheet, create a layer of zucchini slices, a layer of meat sauce, a layer of ricotta mixture, and repeat until you run out of ingredients. Finish with a layer of ricotta mixture. Cover the pan with aluminum foil and cook in the oven for 20-25 minutes, then uncover and cook for a further 10 minutes or until the courgette lasagna is well cooked and the cheese is golden. Serve the Zucchini Lasagna with Ricotta and Meat Sauce hot.

PORCINI MUSHROOM RISOTTO WITH PARMESAN

Preparation Times: 10-15 minutes

Cooking Times: 20-25 minutes

Doses Ingredients for 4 People:

320 g of Arborio or Carnaroli rice

200 g fresh or dried porcini mushrooms (soaked)

1 onion, chopped

2 cloves garlic, finely chopped

1/2 cup dry white wine

1.5 liters vegetable or

mushroom broth (hot)

1/2 cup grated parmesan

2 tablespoons butter

Extra virgin olive oil

Salt and black pepper to taste

Chopped fresh parsley (for garnish)

Preparation:

If you are using dried mushrooms, soak them in hot water for about 15-20 minutes, then drain and chop them roughly. In a saucepan, heat some olive oil and add the chopped onion and garlic. Cook until translucent. Add the mushrooms (fresh or dried) and cook until they start to brown. Add the rice and toast it for a few minutes until it becomes slightly transparent. Pour in the white wine and stir until the wine has been absorbed by the rice.

Begin adding the hot broth, one ladle at a time, stirring constantly and waiting for the liquid to be absorbed before adding the next. Continue cooking until the rice is al dente and the risotto has a creamy texture. Turn off the heat and add the grated parmesan and butter. Mix well until you obtain a creamy risotto. Add salt and pepper to taste and garnish with chopped fresh parsley. Serve the Porcini Mushroom Risotto with hot Parmesan.

CHICKEN SALAD WITH AVOCADO AND VEGETABLES

Preparation Times: 15-20 minutes

Cooking Times: 10-15 minutes

Doses Ingredients for 4 People:

For the Salad:

2 cooked chicken breasts and

cut into strips or cubes

2 avocados, cut into cubes

Mixed lettuce or salad a

green leaves to taste

Vegetables to taste (e.g. tomatoes,

cucumbers, carrots, peppers)

Seeds of your choice (e.g. seeds of

sunflower, pumpkin seeds)

Cheese to taste (e.g.

feta cheese, goat cheese)

For the Vinaigrette:

1/4 cup extra virgin olive oil

Juice of 1 lemon

1 teaspoon Dijon mustard

Salt and black pepper to taste

Preparation:

In a large bowl, mix the cooked chicken, avocado, lettuce, greens and seeds. In a jar or small bowl, make the vinaigrette by combining the olive oil, lemon juice, mustard, salt, and pepper. Shake or mix well. Pour the vinaigrette over the salad and toss gently to coat the ingredients in the vinaigrette. Garnish with cheese to taste and serve the Chicken Salad with Avocado and Vegetables as a main course.

BROWN RICE SPAGHETTI WITH ARUGULA PESTO

Preparation Times: 15-20 minutes

Cooking Times: 10-15 minutes (for pasta)

Doses Ingredients for 4 People:

320 g of brown rice spaghetti

2 cups fresh arugula leaves

1/2 cup toasted walnuts

2 cloves garlic, finely chopped

1/2 cup grated Parmesan

1/2 cup extra virgin olive oil

Juice of 1 lemon

Salt and black pepper to taste

Preparation:

Cook brown rice noodles according to package instructions until al dente. Drain and set aside. In a food processor, blend the arugula, toasted walnuts, garlic, grated cheese, lemon juice, salt and pepper. Continue blending while slowly adding the olive oil until you have a creamy pesto. In a large bowl, toss the rice noodles with the arugula pesto until well coated. Serve the Brown Rice Spaghetti with Arugula Pesto hot or at room temperature.

SWEET POTATO OMELETE WITH BACON AND ONION

Preparation Times: 15-20 minutes

Cooking Times: 15-20 minutes

Doses Ingredients for 4 People:

2 medium sweet potatoes, peeled and cut into cubes

100g bacon, diced

1 onion, cut into slices

8 eggs

1/4 cup milk

Salt and black pepper to taste

Extra virgin olive oil

Cheese to taste

(optional, for garnish)

Preparation:

In a non-stick pan, heat some olive oil and add the sweet potato cubes. Cook over medium-low heat until potatoes are tender and lightly browned. Move the potatoes to a plate. In the same pan, add the bacon and cook until crispy. Move the bacon to a plate with paper towels to remove excess oil. In the same pan, add the onion slices and cook until translucent. In a bowl, beat the eggs with the milk, salt and pepper. Add the sweet potatoes, bacon and onion to the beaten eggs and mix well.

Heat some olive oil in the pan, then pour the entire egg, potato, and bacon mixture into the pan. Cook over medium-low heat until the edges of the omelette are golden brown and the inside is completely cooked. You can cover the pan with a lid to aid cooking. If desired, top with cheese to taste and cook until cheese melts. Serve the Sweet Potato Frittata with Bacon and Onion hot or at room temperature.

POTATO GNOCCHI WITH TOMATO SAUCE

Preparation Times: 30-40 minutes

Cooking Times: 5-10 minutes

Doses Ingredients for 4 People:

For the Gnocchi:

500 g of potato gnocchi (you can use them fresh or frozen)

Salt to taste

For the Tomato Sauce:

2 cups tomato puree

2 cloves garlic, finely chopped

1/4 cup fresh basil, chopped

Salt and black pepper to taste

Extra virgin olive oil

Preparation:

In a large saucepan, bring plenty of salted water to a boil. Cook the gnocchi according to package instructions or until they float. Drain the gnocchi and set them aside. In a pan, heat some olive oil and add the minced garlic. Cook until fragrant. Add the tomato puree, fresh basil, salt and pepper. Cook over medium-low heat for about 5-10 minutes or until the sauce thickens slightly. Add the potato gnocchi to the tomato sauce in the pan and mix well to coat. Serve the Potato Gnocchi with Tomato Sauce hot, garnished with fresh basil if desired.

ZUCCHINI TAGLIATELLE WITH LIGHT ALFREDO SAUCE

Preparation Times: 15-20 minutes

Cooking Times: 10-15 minutes

Doses Ingredients for 4 People:

4 medium courgettes, cut into

julienne or with a spiralizer

2 tablespoons light butter

2 cloves garlic, finely chopped

1 cup light cream

1/2 cup grated Parmesan

Nutmeg to taste

Salt and black pepper to taste

Chopped fresh parsley (for garnish)

Preparation:

In a skillet, melt light butter over medium-low heat. Add minced garlic and cook until fragrant. Add the julienned or spiralized courgettes and cook for 2-3 minutes or until tender but still crunchy. Pour the light cream into the pan and mix well. Add the grated Parmesan and continue mixing until you obtain a creamy sauce. Flavor the sauce with a pinch of nutmeg, salt and black pepper to taste. Serve the Zucchini Tagliatelle with Light Alfredo Sauce, garnished with chopped fresh parsley if desired.

QUINOA RISOTTO WITH ASPARAGUS AND CHEESE

Preparation Times: 10-15 minutes

Cooking Times: 20-25 minutes

Doses Ingredients for 4 People:

1 cup quinoa

1 bunch asparagus, cut into small pieces

1 onion, chopped

2 cloves garlic, finely chopped

4 cups vegetable broth (hot)

1 cup Gouda cheese or cheese

grated to taste

2 tablespoons extra virgin olive oil

Salt and black pepper to taste

Preparation:

In a saucepan, heat the olive oil over medium heat. Add the chopped onion and garlic and cook until translucent. Add the quinoa and toast it for about 2 minutes, stirring constantly. Add the chopped asparagus and continue to cook for another couple of minutes. Pour a cup of hot broth into the pot and stir. Continue to cook over medium heat, stirring occasionally. Once the broth has been absorbed, add another cup of broth and repeat the process until the quinoa is cooked (about 15-20 minutes). Add the grated cheese and mix until you obtain a creamy consistency. Season with salt and pepper to taste. Serve the Quinoa Risotto with Asparagus and Cheese, garnishing with cheese to taste if desired.

ZUCCHINI SPAGHETTI WITH LEMON PRAWNS

Preparation Times: 15-20 minutes

Cooking Times: 10-15 minutes

Doses Ingredients for 4 People:

4 medium courgettes, cut into julienne strips

or with a spiralizer

400 g of peeled and cleaned prawns

Juice and grated zest of 1 lemon

3 cloves garlic, finely chopped

2 tablespoons butter

2 tablespoons extra virgin olive oil

Salt and black pepper to taste

Chopped fresh parsley (for garnish)

Preparation:

In a skillet, heat the olive oil and butter over medium heat. Add minced garlic and cook until fragrant. Add the peeled prawns and cook for 2-3 minutes per side or until pink and cooked through. Remove the shrimp from the pan and set aside. In the same pan, add the julienned courgettes and cook for about 2-3 minutes or until tender but still crunchy. Add the lemon juice and grated zest to the courgettes and mix well. Combine the previously cooked prawns with the lemon courgettes, mix and cook for another minute. Season with salt and pepper to taste. Garnish with chopped fresh parsley and serve the Courgette Spaghetti with Lemon Prawns hot.

GRILLED SALMON WITH CAULIFLOWER RISOTTO

Preparation Times: 15-20 minutes

Cooking Times: 20-25 minutes

Doses Ingredients for 4 People:

For the Salmon:

4 salmon fillets

Extra virgin olive oil

Salt and black pepper to taste

Grated lemon zest

(optional, for garnish)

For the Cauliflower Risotto:

1 medium cauliflower, divided into florets

1 onion, chopped

2 cloves garlic, finely chopped

2 cups chicken or vegetable broth (hot)

1/2 cup grated Parmesan

2 tablespoons butter

Salt and black pepper to taste

Preparation:

Preheat grill to medium-high heat. Brush the salmon fillets with a little olive oil and season with salt and pepper. Grill the salmon for about 4-5 minutes per side or until cooked through. You can garnish with grated lemon zest before serving. Meanwhile, steam the cauliflower florets until tender (about 5-7 minutes). Then blend the steamed florets in a food processor until they have a rice-like consistency.

In a skillet, melt the butter over medium-low heat. Add the chopped onion and cook until translucent. Add the minced garlic and cook for a minute until fragrant. Add the cauliflower "rice" and stir for about 2-3 minutes. Pour the hot broth gradually into the cauliflower "rice", stirring constantly until the broth is absorbed and the risotto becomes creamy (about 10-15 minutes). Remove from the heat, add the grated Parmesan cheese and mix until you get a creamy consistency. Season with salt and pepper to taste. Serve grilled salmon with hot cauliflower risotto.

WHOLE WHOLE SPAGHETTI WITH FRESH TOMATO SAUCE

Preparation Times: 15-20 minutes

Cooking Times: 20-25 minutes

Doses Ingredients for 4 People:

320 g of wholemeal spaghetti

4 ripe tomatoes, cut into cubes

2 cloves garlic, finely chopped

1/4 cup fresh basil, chopped

2 tablespoons extra virgin olive oil

Salt and black pepper to taste

Grated Parmesan cheese

(optional, for garnish)

Preparation:

Cook wholemeal spaghetti in a pan of salted water following package instructions until al dente. Drain the pasta and set it aside. In a skillet, heat the olive oil over medium heat. Add minced garlic and cook until fragrant. Add the tomato cubes and cook for about 10-15 minutes or until the tomatoes soften and release their juices. Add fresh basil, salt and pepper. Mix well. Add the whole-wheat spaghetti to the fresh tomato sauce in the pan and stir until well coated. Serve Wholemeal Spaghetti with Fresh Tomato Sauce hot, garnished with grated Parmesan cheese if desired.

PASTA SALAD WITH GRILLED VEGETABLES

Preparation Times: 15-20 minutes

Cooking Times: 10-15 minutes

Doses Ingredients for 4 People:

300 g pasta of your choice (penne, farfalle, or other short pasta)

2 cups mixed vegetables (zucchini, peppers, aubergines, tomatoes) cut into slices or cubes

2 tablespoons extra virgin olive oil

Salt and black pepper to taste

1/4 cup fresh basil, chopped

1/4 cup feta cheese, crumbled

1/4 cup black olives, pitted and cut into rounds (optional)

Preparation:

Cook the pasta in a pot of salted water following the package instructions until al dente. Drain the pasta, rinse it under cold water and set it aside. While the pasta cools, you can grill the vegetables. Brush the vegetables with olive oil and grill them on a grill or in a grill pan until tender and lightly browned. Season with salt and pepper to taste. In a large bowl, combine the cooled pasta and grilled vegetables. Mix well. Add fresh basil, feta cheese, and black olives (if using). Mix again. Serve the Pasta Salad with Grilled Vegetables at room temperature or cold.

SPELLED RISOTTO WITH MUSHROOMS AND PARMESAN

Preparation Times: 15-20 minutes

Cooking Times: 30-35 minutes

Doses Ingredients for 4 People:

1 cup pearled spelled

250 g of mixed mushrooms (e.g. champignons, porcini mushrooms), sliced meats

1 onion, chopped

2 cloves garlic, finely chopped

1/2 cup dry white wine

4 cups vegetable broth (hot)

1/2 cup grated Parmesan

2 tablespoons extra virgin olive oil

Salt and black pepper to taste

Chopped fresh parsley (for garnish)

Preparation:

In a saucepan, heat the olive oil over medium heat. Add the chopped onion and garlic and cook until translucent. Add the sliced mushrooms and cook until they release their liquid and turn golden. Add the pearled spelled and toast it for about 2 minutes, stirring constantly. Pour the white wine into the pan and cook until it has evaporated. Start adding the vegetable broth, one ladle at a time, stirring constantly and waiting for the broth to be absorbed before adding more. Continue this process until the spelled is cooked and has reached a creamy consistency (about 30-35 minutes). Add the grated Parmesan cheese and mix until you obtain an even creamier consistency. Season with salt and pepper to taste. Garnish with fresh chopped parsley and serve the Spelled Risotto with Mushrooms and Parmesan hot.

CHICKEN CACCIATORA WITH WHOLE BARLEY

Preparation Times: 20-25 minutes

Cooking Times: 45-50 minutes

Doses Ingredients for 4 People:

4 chicken thighs or chicken breasts (with

or skinless, your choice)

1 onion, chopped

2 cloves garlic, finely chopped

1 red pepper, cut into strips

1 green pepper, cut into strips

1 cup peeled tomatoes, chopped

1/2 cup dry red wine

1 cup whole grain barley

2 cups chicken broth (hot)

2 tablespoons extra virgin olive oil

1 teaspoon dried oregano

1 teaspoon dried rosemary

Salt and black pepper to taste

Chopped fresh parsley (for garnish)

Preparation:

In a large pot or saucepan, heat the olive oil over medium-high heat. Add the chicken and brown until golden on both sides. Transfer the chicken to a plate and set aside. In the same pot, add the onion, garlic and peppers. Cook for about 5 minutes or until the vegetables are tender. Add the peeled tomatoes, red wine, oregano, rosemary, salt and pepper. Return chicken to pot.

Cover the pot and cook over medium-low heat for about 30 to 35 minutes or until the chicken is cooked through and tender. Meanwhile, cook the whole barley in another pot according to the package instructions. Drain it and set it aside. When the chicken is done, remove it from the pot and set aside. Add the cooked whole grain barley to the sauce in the pot and mix well. Serve the Chicken Cacciatora with Whole Barley hot, garnished with fresh chopped parsley if desired.

WHOLE WHOLE PAPPARDELLE WITH BOLOGNESE SAUCE

Preparation Times: 20-25 minutes

Cooking Times: 45-50 minutes

Doses Ingredients for 4 People:

320 g of wholemeal pappardelle

400g lean minced meat

(beef, pork or mixed)

1 onion, chopped

2 carrots, chopped

2 celery sticks, chopped

2 cloves garlic, finely chopped

1 cup peeled tomatoes, chopped

1/2 cup dry red wine

2 tablespoons extra virgin olive oil

1 teaspoon dried oregano

1 teaspoon dried basil

Salt and black pepper to taste

Preparation:

In a large pot, heat the olive oil over medium heat. Add the chopped onion, carrots and celery and cook for about 5-7 minutes or until the vegetables are tender. Add the minced garlic and cook for a minute until fragrant. Add the minced meat and cook until golden brown and fully cooked. Pour the red wine into the pot and cook until it has evaporated. Add the peeled tomatoes, oregano, basil, salt and pepper. Reduce the heat and let simmer for about 30-35 minutes, stirring occasionally.

Meanwhile, cook the wholemeal pappardelle in a pan of salted water following the package instructions until al dente. Drain the pasta and set it aside. When the Bolognese sauce is ready, add the pappardelle to the sauce in the pan and mix well to blend the flavors. Serve wholemeal Pappardelle with Bolognese sauce hot.

QUINOA SALAD WITH CHICKPEAS AND PEPPERS

Preparation Times: 20-25 minutes

Cooking Times: 15-20 minutes

Doses Ingredients for 4 People:

1 cup quinoa

1 can chickpeas, drained and rinsed

2 peppers (one red and one yellow)

cut into cubes

1/2 red onion, finely chopped

1/4 cup fresh parsley, chopped

1/4 cup extra virgin olive oil

Juice of 1 lemon

Salt and black pepper to taste

Preparation:

Rinse the quinoa well under cold running water. Cook the quinoa according to the package instructions. Let cool. In a large bowl, combine the cooked quinoa, chickpeas, bell peppers, red onion and fresh parsley. In a small bowl, prepare the vinaigrette by combining the olive oil, lemon juice, salt, and pepper. Mix well. Pour the vinaigrette over the quinoa salad and mix until all the ingredients are well coated. Serve the Quinoa Salad with Chickpeas and Peppers at room temperature or cold.

BUCKWHEAT SPAGHETTI WITH SPINACH PESTO

Preparation Times: 15-20 minutes

Cooking Times: 10-15 minutes

Doses Ingredients for 4 People:

320 g of buckwheat spaghetti

200 g of fresh spinach

2 cloves garlic, finely chopped

1/2 cup walnuts or pine nuts, toasted

1/2 cup grated Parmesan

1/2 cup extra virgin olive oil

Salt and black pepper to taste

Grated zest of 1 lemon

(optional, for garnish)

Preparation:

Cook the buckwheat spaghetti in a pan of salted water following package instructions until al dente. Drain the pasta and set it aside. In a pan, heat some olive oil over medium heat. Add fresh spinach and cook until soft and wilted. In a blender, combine cooked spinach, minced garlic, toasted walnuts or pine nuts, grated Parmesan cheese, and extra virgin olive oil. Blend until you get a smooth pesto. Season with salt and pepper to taste. Combine the spinach pesto with the buckwheat spaghetti and mix until well coated. Serve Buckwheat Spaghetti with Spinach Pesto hot, garnishing with grated lemon zest if desired.

BARLEY RISOTTO WITH COURGETTES AND PEPPERS

Preparation Times: 20-25 minutes

Cooking Times: 30-35 minutes

Doses Ingredients for 4 People:

1 cup pearl barley

2 medium courgettes, diced

1 red pepper, diced

1 onion, chopped

2 cloves garlic, finely chopped

4 cups vegetable broth (hot)

1/2 cup dry white wine

2 tablespoons extra virgin olive oil

1/2 cup grated Parmesan

Salt and black pepper to taste

Chopped fresh parsley (for garnish)

Preparation:

In a saucepan, heat the olive oil over medium heat. Add the chopped onion and garlic and cook until translucent. Add the diced courgettes and bell pepper and cook for about 5-7 minutes or until the vegetables are tender. Add the pearl barley and toast for about 2 minutes, stirring constantly. Pour the white wine into the pan and cook until it has evaporated. Start adding the vegetable broth, one ladle at a time, stirring constantly and waiting for the broth to be absorbed before adding more. Continue this process until the orzo is cooked and has reached a creamy consistency (about 30-35 minutes). Add the grated Parmesan cheese and mix until you obtain an even creamier consistency. Season with salt and pepper to taste. Garnish with fresh chopped parsley and serve the Barley Risotto with Courgettes and Peppers hot.

EGG OMELETE WITH BACON AND POTATOES

Preparation Times: 15-20 minutes

Cooking Times: 15-20 minutes

Doses Ingredients for 4 People:

8 eggs

100g smoked bacon, diced

2 medium potatoes, peeled and

cut into thin slices

1 onion, chopped

2 tablespoons extra virgin olive oil

Salt and black pepper to taste

Grated cheese

(optional, for garnish)

Chopped fresh parsley (for garnish)

Preparation:

In a nonstick skillet, heat the olive oil over medium heat. Add the sliced potatoes and cook until soft and lightly browned. Drain them and set them aside. In the same pan, add the diced bacon and cook until crisp. Drain it and set it aside. In a bowl, beat the eggs and add the chopped onion, cooked potatoes and crispy bacon. Mix well and add salt and pepper to taste. Heat the non-stick pan and pour in the egg, potato and bacon mixture. Cook over medium-low heat for about 10 to 15 minutes or until the bottom is golden brown and the top is almost completely set. To cook the top, you can place the pan under the grill in your preheated oven for a few minutes, but be careful not to let it burn. Cut the omelette into wedges and serve hot.

LENTIL SPAGHETTI WITH TOMATO SAUCE

Preparation Times: 15-20 minutes

Cooking Times: 20-25 minutes

Doses Ingredients for 4 People:

320 g of lentil spaghetti

(or other lentil-based pasta)

2 cups tomato sauce

2 cloves garlic, finely chopped

1 onion, chopped

2 tablespoons extra virgin olive oil

1 teaspoon dried oregano

Salt and black pepper to taste

Grated Parmesan (for garnish)

Fresh basil (for garnish)

Preparation:

In a saucepan, heat the olive oil over medium heat. Add the chopped onion and garlic and cook until translucent. Add the tomato sauce and dried oregano. Cook over medium-low heat for about 15-20 minutes, stirring occasionally. Season with salt and pepper to taste. Meanwhile, cook the lentil spaghetti in a pan of salted water according to package instructions until al dente. Drain the pasta. Combine the lentil spaghetti with the tomato sauce and mix well to combine the flavours. Serve the Lentil Spaghetti with Tomato Sauce hot, garnished with grated Parmesan cheese and fresh basil leaves.

PIZZA WITH CAULIFLOWER CRUST

Preparation Times: 20-25 minutes

Cooking Times: 30-35 minutes

Doses Ingredients for 4 People:

For the Cauliflower Crust:

1 small cauliflower, cleaned and chopped finely or grated

1 egg

1 cup grated mozzarella cheese

1 teaspoon dried oregano

Salt and black pepper to taste

For the seasoning:

1/2 cup tomato sauce

Grated mozzarella cheese to taste

Topping of your choice (e.g. sliced tomatoes, olives,

mushrooms, peppers, fresh basil, etc.)

Preparation:

Preheat the oven to 200°C and place a baking tray with parchment paper. In a bowl, combine the chopped or grated cauliflower, egg, grated mozzarella cheese, dried oregano, salt and pepper. Mix until you obtain a homogeneous mixture. Transfer the dough to the prepared baking sheet and spread it out evenly to form a thin crust. Place the cauliflower crust in the oven and bake for about 15-20 minutes or until golden brown. Remove crust from oven and add tomato sauce, shredded mozzarella cheese and desired toppings. Place the pizza back in the oven and cook for another 10-15 minutes or until the cheese is melted and golden. Remove the pizza from the oven, cut it into slices and serve hot.

AUBERGINE LASAGNE WITH RICOTTA AND SPINACH

Preparation Times: 30-35 minutes

Cooking Times: 45-50 minutes

Doses Ingredients for 4 People:

2 medium aubergines, cut into thin slices

1 pack of dry lasagna

2 cups cottage cheese

2 cups fresh spinach or baby spinach

frozen, cooked and well squeezed

1 cup grated mozzarella cheese

1/2 cup grated Parmesan

1 egg

2 cups tomato sauce

2 cloves garlic, finely chopped

Salt and black pepper to taste

Chopped fresh parsley (for garnish)

Preparation:

Preheat the oven to 180°C and place a baking tray. In a pan, heat some olive oil and cook the aubergine slices until soft and lightly browned. Drain them on absorbent paper and set them aside. In a bowl, mix the ricotta, cooked and squeezed spinach, grated mozzarella cheese, grated Parmesan cheese, egg, chopped garlic, salt and pepper. Start assembling the lasagna one layer at a time:

starts with a layer of tomato sauce, followed by alternating layers of dry lasagna, aubergine slices and the ricotta and spinach mixture. Repeat until the ingredients are used up, making sure the last layer is cheese and salsada. Cover the pan with aluminum foil and bake in the oven for about 35-40 minutes. Remove the foil and cook for a further 10-15 minutes or until the surface is golden and the lasagne is cooked. Garnish with chopped fresh parsley and let rest for a few minutes before serving.

PUMPKIN GNOCCHI WITH BUTTER AND SAGE

Preparation Times: 30-35 minutes

Cooking Times: 10-15 minutes

Doses Ingredients for 4 People:

500 g of pumpkin gnocchi (available commercially available or homemade)

100 g of butter

Fresh sage leaves (about 10-12 leaves)

Salt and black pepper to taste

Grated Parmesan cheese (optional, for garnish)

Preparation:

Bring a pan of lightly salted water to a boil. Meanwhile, in a large skillet, melt the butter over medium heat. Add the fresh sage leaves and cook until the butter starts to turn golden and the sage leaves are crispy. Remove the sage and set aside. Cook the pumpkin gnocchi in boiling water according to package instructions or until they rise to the surface (usually takes only a few minutes). Drain them with a slotted spoon and transfer them to the pan with the butter and sage. Sauté the gnocchi in the pan for a few minutes until they are well coated in the flavored butter. Season with salt and pepper to taste. Serve the Pumpkin Gnocchi with Butter and Sage hot, garnishing with grated Parmesan cheese if desired.

POLENTA WITH MUSHROOMS AND CHEESE

Preparation Times: 20-25 minutes

Cooking Times: 30-35 minutes

Doses Ingredients for 4 People:

1 cup cornmeal for polenta

4 cups mushroom broth or vegetable broth

250g mixed mushrooms, cut into slices

1 onion, chopped

2 cloves garlic, finely chopped

1 cup cheese to taste), cut into cubes

2 tablespoons extra virgin olive oil

Salt and black pepper to taste

Chopped fresh parsley (for garnish)

Preparation:

In a saucepan, bring mushroom broth or vegetable broth to a boil. Pour the corn flour into the pan, stirring constantly to avoid the formation of lumps. Reduce the heat and cook the polenta over low heat for about 25-30 minutes, stirring occasionally, until it becomes thick and creamy. Meanwhile, in a skillet, heat the olive oil over medium heat. Add the chopped onion and cook until translucent. Add the chopped garlic cloves and sliced mushrooms. Cook until mushrooms are golden and tender. Season with salt and pepper to taste. When the polenta is ready, turn off the heat and add the cheese of your choice. Stir until the cheese has completely melted into the polenta. Serve the Polenta with Mushrooms and Cheese hot, garnished with fresh chopped parsley.

CARROT SPAGHETTI WITH BASIL PESTO

Preparation Times: 20-25 minutes

Cooking Times: 10-15 minutes

Doses Ingredients for 4 People:

320 g of carrot spaghetti (available in commercial or homemade)

For the Basil Pesto:

2 cups fresh basil leaves

1/2 cup toasted walnuts or pine nuts

2 cloves garlic, finely chopped

1/2 cup extra virgin olive oil

1/2 cup grated Parmesan

Salt and black pepper to taste

Lemon juice (optional, for freshness)

Preparation:

Cook the carrot spaghetti in a pot of salted water according to package instructions or until al dente. Drain the pasta and set it aside. Meanwhile, make the basil pesto: In a blender, combine fresh basil leaves, toasted walnuts or pine nuts, minced garlic, grated Parmigiano-Reggiano cheese, and extra virgin olive oil. Blend until you get a smooth pesto. Season with salt and pepper to taste and, if desired, add a little lemon juice for freshness. Combine the basil pesto with the carrot spaghetti and mix until well coated. Serve the Carrot Spaghetti with Basil Pesto hot.

RECIPES
SECOND DISHES

GRILLED CHICKEN FILLET WITH AVOCADO SAUCE

Preparation time: 15 minutes

Cooking time: 10-12 minutes

Doses: 4 people

Ingredients:

4 chicken fillets

Salt and pepper to taste

Extra virgin olive oil to taste

1 ripe avocado

Juice of 1 lime

1 clove of garlic

Chopped fresh coriander

Salt and pepper to taste

Preparation:

Marinate the meat: In a bowl, season the chicken fillets with salt, pepper and a drizzle of oil. Leave to marinate for at least 15 minutes. Grill the chicken: Heat the grill and cook the fillets for about 5-6 minutes per side, or until cooked through. Prepare the sauce: Meanwhile, in a bowl, mash the avocado with a fork. Add the lime juice, minced garlic, coriander and season with salt and pepper. Serve: Serve the grilled chicken with the avocado salsa. You can accompany it with a mixed salad or baked potatoes.

BAKED SALMON WITH PISTACHIO CRUST

Preparation time: 20 minutes

Cooking time: 20-25 minutes

Doses: 4 people

Ingredients:

4 salmon steaks

50g unsalted pistachios

Breadcrumbs to taste

Chopped parsley

Garlic powder

Salt and pepper to taste

Extra virgin olive oil to taste

Lemon

Preparation:

Prepare the crust: In a shallow dish, coarsely chop the pistachios. Add the breadcrumbs, chopped parsley, garlic powder, salt and pepper. Bread the salmon: Season the salmon steaks with salt, pepper and a drizzle of oil. Pass them in the pistachio breading, pressing lightly to make them adhere. Cook in the oven: Place the salmon steaks on a baking tray lined with baking paper and cook in a preheated oven at 200°C for approximately 20-25 minutes, or until the salmon is cooked and the crust is golden. Serve: Serve the salmon with a slice of lemon. Accompany with steamed vegetables or a salad.

BEEF STEAK WITH MUSHROOM SAUCE

Preparation Times: 10 minutes

Cooking Times: 15-20 minutes

Doses Ingredients for 4 People:

4 beef steaks (about 200-250 g each)

Salt and black pepper to taste

Extra virgin olive oil

For the Mushroom Sauce:

200 g of mushrooms (porcini, champignons or other mushrooms of your choice), sliced

2 cloves garlic, finely chopped

1/2 cup beef broth

2 tablespoons butter

Chopped fresh parsley for garnish

Preparation:

Preheat a nonstick skillet over medium-high heat. Brush the beef steaks lightly with olive oil and season with salt and black pepper to taste. Cook the steaks on the preheated skillet for 3 to 4 minutes per side for medium-rare, or longer if you prefer your meat rarer. Remove the steaks from the pan and let them rest. In the same pan, add the butter and minced garlic. Cook the garlic for a minute until fragrant. Add the sliced mushrooms and cook until golden and tender. Pour the meat broth into the pan with the mushrooms and bring everything to the boil. Reduce heat and simmer over medium-low heat until sauce reduces slightly and thickens. Serve the beef steaks hot, spooning the mushroom sauce over them and garnishing with chopped fresh parsley.

STEAMED TILAPIA FILLET WITH VEGETABLES

Preparation Times: 15 minutes

Cooking Times: 15-20 minutes

Doses Ingredients for 4 People:

4 tilapia fillets (about 150 g each)

Salt and black pepper to taste

1 lemon, cut into thin slices

For the Steamed Vegetables:

400 g of a mix of vegetables to taste (broccoli, carrots, courgettes, etc.), cut into pieces

Juice of 1 lemon

Extra virgin olive oil

Chopped fresh parsley for garnish

Preparation:

Preheat a steamer. Season the tilapia fillets with salt, black pepper and lemon juice. Arrange the tilapia fillets on glass kitchen plates, add lemon slices to each fillet. Place the vegetable pieces in the steamer and steam for 8 to 10 minutes or until the vegetables are tender but still crunchy. Meanwhile, heat a nonstick skillet over medium-high heat and brush lightly with olive oil. Cook tilapia fillets for 2 to 3 minutes per side or until meat is opaque and flakes easily with a fork. Serve the steamed tilapia fillets with the vegetables, garnished with chopped fresh parsley and additional lemon slices, if desired.

ROAST CHICKEN WITH AVOCADO SAUCE

Preparation Times: 15 minutes

Cooking Times: 30-40 minutes

Doses Ingredients for 4 People:

4 skinless, boneless chicken breasts

Salt and black pepper to taste

Extra virgin olive oil

For the Avocado Sauce:

2 ripe avocados

Juice of 1 lime

2 cloves garlic, finely chopped

1/4 cup fresh coriander leaves

1/4 cup Greek yogurt

Salt and black pepper to taste

Preparation:

Preheat the oven to 190°C. Season the chicken breasts with salt, black pepper and a drizzle of olive oil. Place the chicken breasts on a baking sheet and bake in the preheated oven for 30 to 40 minutes or until the chicken is browned and cooked through. While the chicken cooks, make the avocado salsa. In a blender, combine peeled avocados, lime juice, minced garlic, fresh cilantro, Greek yogurt, salt, and black pepper. Blend until smooth. Serve the roasted chicken hot, with a generous dollop of avocado salsa on top of each chicken breast.

GRILLED PRAWNS WITH GARLIC BUTTER

Preparation Times: 15 minutes

Cooking Times: 5-7 minutes

Doses Ingredients for 4 People:

16 extra large prawns, peeled and cleaned

Salt and black pepper to taste

Extra virgin olive oil

For the Garlic Butter:

1/2 cup butter, softened

4 cloves garlic, finely chopped

Chopped fresh parsley for garnish

Grated lemon zest

Preparation:

Preheat an outdoor grill or kitchen grill to medium-high heat. Season the prawns with salt, black pepper and a drizzle of olive oil. In a small bowl, mix the softened butter with the minced garlic. Grill the prawns for 2-3 minutes per side or until pink and lightly browned. During the last few minutes of cooking, brush the prawns with the garlic butter and cook for an additional minute to allow the butter to adhere. Serve the grilled prawns hot, garnished with chopped fresh parsley and grated lemon zest.

BAKED PORK RIBS WITH SPICE RUB

Preparation Times: 15 minutes

Cooking Times: 2-2.5 hours

Doses Ingredients for 4 People:

2 kg of pork ribs

Salt and black pepper to taste

For the Spice Rub:

2 tablespoons smoked paprika

1 tablespoon black pepper

1 tablespoon of salt

1 tablespoon brown sugar

1 teaspoon sweet paprika

1 teaspoon cumin powder

1/2 teaspoon cayenne pepper

(optional for a spicy touch)

Preparation:

Preheat the oven to 150°C. In a bowl, mix all the ingredients for the Spice Rub. Prepare the pork ribs, removing any membranes and excess fat. Season the ribs on both sides with salt and black pepper. Generously sprinkle the Spice Rub over the pork ribs, making sure to cover both sides evenly. Wrap the ribs in cling film and let them marinate in the refrigerator for at least 30 minutes or preferably several hours. Place the marinated ribs on a baking sheet and cover them with aluminum foil. Cook in the preheated oven for 2 to 2.5 hours or until the ribs are tender and fall easily from the bones. During the last 15-20 minutes of cooking, you can uncover the ribs to brown them slightly. Once cooked, serve the Baked Pork Ribs hot.

CHICKEN CURRY WITH COCONUT MILK

Preparation Times: 15 minutes

Cooking Times: 25-30 minutes

Doses Ingredients for 4 People:

500g chicken breast, cut into cubes

Salt and black pepper to taste

2 tablespoons vegetable oil

1 onion, chopped

3 cloves garlic, finely chopped

2 tablespoons red or green curry paste (depending on your preferences)

1 can of coconut milk (about 400 ml)

2 tablespoons fish sauce

1 tablespoon brown sugar

Juice of 1 lime

Fresh basil leaves for garnish

Preparation:

Season the chicken breast cubes with salt and black pepper. In a large skillet, heat the vegetable oil over medium-high heat. Add the chopped onion and minced garlic and cook until golden and fragrant. Add the red or green curry paste to the pan and stir for about a minute to toast it and release its flavors. Add the chicken cubes and cook until golden on all sides. Pour the coconut milk into the pan and bring everything to a boil. Reduce heat and simmer over medium-low heat for 15 to 20 minutes or until chicken is cooked through and sauce has thickened. Add the fish sauce, brown sugar, and lime juice to the pan. Mix well and cook for another 2-3 minutes. Serve the Chicken Curry with Coconut Milk hot, garnished with fresh basil leaves.

FRENCH SOLE WITH BUTTER AND PARSLEY

Preparation Times: 15 minutes

Cooking Times: 10-15 minutes

Doses Ingredients for 4 People:

4 sole fillets

Salt and black pepper to taste

1/2 cup flour

2 eggs, beaten

2 tablespoons butter

2 tablespoons of olive oil

Juice of 1 lemon

2 tablespoons chopped fresh parsley

Preparation:

Season the sole fillets with salt and black pepper. Dredge each sole fillet in flour, making sure it is evenly coated, then dip it in the beaten eggs. In a large nonstick skillet, heat the butter and olive oil over medium-high heat. Cook the sole fillets in the pan for about 2-3 minutes per side or until golden and crispy. Squeeze lemon juice over the sole fillets and sprinkle with chopped fresh parsley before serving.

TURKEY BREAST STUFFED WITH SPINACH AND CHEESE

Preparation Times: 20 minutes

Cooking Times: 25-30 minutes

Doses Ingredients for 4 People:

4 turkey breasts, boned and skinless

Salt and black pepper to taste

2 cups fresh spinach, chopped

1 cup grated cheese to taste

(cheddar, mozzarella, or anything else of your choice)

2 cloves garlic, finely chopped

2 tablespoons of olive oil

1/2 cup chicken broth

1 glass of dry white wine (optional)

Preparation:

Pre-heat the oven to 180°C. Season the turkey breasts with salt and black pepper. Open each turkey breast to form a pocket. In a skillet, heat the olive oil over medium heat. Add the minced garlic and cook for a minute until fragrant. Add the chopped spinach and cook until wilted. Remove the pan from the heat and mix the spinach with the grated cheese. Stuff each turkey breast with the spinach and cheese mixture. Place the stuffed turkey breasts in a baking dish and pour the chicken broth (and white wine, if using) into the baking dish. Cover the baking dish with foil and bake in the preheated oven for 25 to 30 minutes or until the turkey is cooked through. Serve the Stuffed Turkey Breasts with Spinach and Cheese hot, accompanied with the cooking sauce if desired.

CHICKEN MEATBALLS WITH TOMATO SAUCE

Preparation Times: 20 minutes

Cooking Times: 20-25 minutes

Doses Ingredients for 4 People:

500g minced chicken breast

1/2 cup breadcrumbs

1/4 cup grated Parmesan

1 egg

1 clove garlic, finely chopped

Salt and black pepper to taste

For the Tomato Sauce:

1 can (400 g) peeled tomatoes

1/2 onion, chopped

2 cloves garlic, finely chopped

1 tablespoon olive oil

Salt and black pepper to taste

Fresh basil for garnish

Preparation:

In a bowl, mix the ground chicken breast, breadcrumbs, Parmesan cheese, egg, minced garlic, salt and black pepper. Mix well until you obtain a homogeneous mixture. With wet hands, shape the mixture into small meatballs. In a nonstick skillet, heat the olive oil over medium heat. Add the meatballs and cook until golden brown on all sides and cooked through, about 20-25 minutes.

Meanwhile, prepare the tomato sauce. In a pan, heat the olive oil and add the chopped onion and garlic. Cook until golden and fragrant. Add the peeled tomatoes to the pan and mash them with a fork. Cook over medium-low heat for 10 to 15 minutes or until sauce has thickened. Season with salt and black pepper to taste. Serve the chicken meatballs hot, with the tomato sauce on top and garnished with fresh basil.

GRILLED TUNA WITH BLACK OLIVE SAUCE

Preparation Times: 15 minutes

Cooking Times: 5-7 minutes

Doses Ingredients for 4 People:

4 fresh tuna fillets

Salt and black pepper to taste

For the Black Olive Sauce:

1/2 cup pitted black olives, chopped

2 tablespoons capers, chopped

2 tablespoons fresh parsley, chopped

2 cloves garlic, finely chopped

Juice of 1 lemon

3 tablespoons extra virgin olive oil

Preparation:

Season the tuna fillets with salt and black pepper. In a bowl, mix the chopped black olives, capers, chopped fresh parsley, minced garlic, lemon juice and extra virgin olive oil to make the sauce. Preheat an outdoor grill or kitchen grill to high heat. Grill the tuna fillets for 2-3 minutes per side or until cooked to perfection and have a light golden crust on the outside. Serve the grilled tuna hot, with a generous dollop of black olive sauce on top of each fillet.

PORK CURRY WITH BROCCOLI

Preparation Times: 15 minutes

Cooking Times: 20-25 minutes

Doses Ingredients for 4 People:

500g diced pork

Salt and black pepper to taste

2 tablespoons of olive oil

1 onion, chopped

2 cloves garlic, finely chopped

2 tablespoons curry paste (of your choice between red, green or yellow)

400ml coconut milk

2 cups broccoli, cut into florets

Juice of 1 lime

Fresh basil for garnish

Preparation:

Season the pork pieces with salt and black pepper. In a large skillet, heat the olive oil over medium heat. Add the chopped onion and minced garlic and cook until golden and fragrant. Add the pork pieces to the pan and cook until browned on all sides. Add the curry paste and mix well with the meat and onions. Pour the coconut milk into the pan and bring everything to a boil. Reduce heat and simmer over medium-low heat for 10 to 15 minutes or until meat is cooked and sauce has thickened. Meanwhile, in a separate pot, steam the broccoli until tender but still crunchy. Add the cooked broccoli to the pork curry and cook for an additional 2-3 minutes. Squeeze lime juice over the dish before serving and garnish with fresh basil leaves.

CHICKEN WITH CASHEW SAUCE AND VEGETABLES

Preparation Times: 15 minutes

Cooking Times: 15-20 minutes

Doses Ingredients for 4 People:

4 chicken breasts, cut into slices or cubes

Salt and black pepper to taste

1 tablespoon olive oil

1 onion, chopped

2 cloves garlic, finely chopped

1 red bell pepper, cut into thin strips

1 green pepper, cut into thin strips

1 cup unsalted cashews, toasted

1 cup coconut milk

2 tablespoons soy sauce

2 tablespoons of brown sugar

Preparation:

Season the chicken slices with salt and black pepper. In a large skillet, heat the olive oil over medium heat. Add the chopped onion and minced garlic and cook until golden and fragrant. Add the red and green pepper strips to the pan and cook until tender. Toast the cashews in a separate pan until golden and crispy. Keep aside. Add the chicken slices to the pan with the vegetables and cook until fully cooked. In a separate bowl, mix the coconut milk, soy sauce, and brown sugar. Pour this mixture into the pan with the chicken and vegetables. Add the toasted cashews to the pan and cook for an additional 2-3 minutes or until the sauce has thickened slightly. Serve the Chicken with Cashew and Vegetable Sauce hot, garnished with fresh basil.

SALMON STEAK WITH PESTO SAUCE

Preparation Times: 10 minutes

Cooking Times: 10-15 minutes

Doses Ingredients for 4 People:

4 salmon steaks

Salt and black pepper to taste

2 tablespoons of olive oil

For the Pesto Sauce:

2 cups fresh basil leaves

1/2 cup grated Parmesan

1/2 cup walnuts or pine nuts

2 cloves garlic, minced

1/2 cup extra virgin olive oil

Salt and black pepper to taste

Preparation:

Season the salmon steaks with salt, black pepper and a little olive oil. Preheat an outdoor grill or kitchen grill to medium-high heat. Grill the salmon steaks for 4 to 5 minutes per side or until cooked through and have a light golden crust on the outside. Meanwhile, make the Pesto Sauce: In a blender, combine the fresh basil, Parmesan cheese, walnuts or pine nuts, minced garlic, extra virgin olive oil, salt, and black pepper. Blend until smooth. Serve the grilled salmon steaks hot, with the Pesto Sauce on top.

GRILLED LAMB RIBS WITH MINT SAUCE

Preparation Times: 15 minutes

Cooking Times: 15-20 minutes

Doses Ingredients for 4 People:

16 lamb ribs

Salt and black pepper to taste

For the Mint Sauce:

1/2 cup fresh mint leaves

1/4 cup Greek yogurt

2 tablespoons lemon juice

2 tablespoons of olive oil

Salt and black pepper to taste

Preparation:

Season the lamb chops with salt and black pepper. Preheat an outdoor grill or kitchen grill to medium-high heat. Grill the lamb ribs for 5-7 minutes per side or until cooked to your preferred doneness (medium rare, medium or well done). Meanwhile, make the Mint Sauce: In a blender, combine the fresh mint leaves, Greek yogurt, lemon juice, olive oil, salt, and black pepper. Blend until smooth. Serve the grilled lamb ribs hot, with the mint sauce on top.

EGG OMELETE WITH BACON AND MUSHROOMS

Preparation Times: 10 minutes

Cooking Times: 15-20 minutes

Doses Ingredients for 4 People:

8 eggs

100 g diced bacon

200g fresh mushrooms, sliced

1 onion, chopped

2 tablespoons of olive oil

Salt and black pepper to taste

Grated Parmesan a

pleasure (optional)

Chopped fresh parsley

for garnish (optional)

Preparation:

In a nonstick skillet, heat the olive oil over medium heat. Add the diced bacon and cook until crispy. Add the chopped onion and sliced mushrooms to the pan and cook until the mushrooms are tender and the onion is golden. In a bowl, beat the eggs with salt and black pepper. Pour the beaten eggs onto the pan with the bacon, mushrooms and onion. Cook over medium-low heat until the eggs are almost completely set. If desired, sprinkle the omelette with grated cheese and place it under the oven grill at 180°C until the cheese is melted and lightly golden. Serve the omelette hot, garnished with fresh chopped parsley if you prefer.

ROSEMARY CHICKEN WHITE WINE SAUCE

Preparation Times: 15 minutes

Cooking Times: 25-30 minutes

Doses Ingredients for 4 People:

4 chicken breasts

Salt and black pepper to taste

2 tablespoons of olive oil

2 sprigs of fresh rosemary

1/2 cup dry white wine

1/2 cup chicken broth

2 tablespoons butter

Chopped fresh parsley

for garnish (optional)

Preparation:

Season the chicken breasts with salt and black pepper. In a large skillet, heat the olive oil over medium-high heat. Add the chicken breasts and brown until golden on both sides. Add fresh rosemary sprigs to the pan. Pour the white wine into the pan and cook over medium heat until the wine has reduced by half. Add the chicken stock and let cook over medium-low heat for about 10 to 15 minutes or until the chicken is fully cooked and the sauce has thickened slightly. Add the butter to the pan and stir until it has melted into the sauce. Serve the rosemary chicken with the warm white wine sauce, garnished with chopped fresh parsley if desired.

SPICY PRAWNS WITH CHILI SAUCE

Preparation Times: 15 minutes

Cooking Times: 5-7 minutes

Doses Ingredients for 4 People:

500 g of peeled and cleaned prawns

Salt and black pepper to taste

2 tablespoons of olive oil

2 cloves garlic, finely chopped

1 fresh red chilli, chopped

(add more or less depending on

your preferred spiciness level)

Juice of 1 lime

Chopped fresh parsley

for garnish (optional)

Preparation:

Season the shrimp with salt and black pepper. In a large skillet, heat the olive oil over medium-high heat. Add the minced garlic and chopped red pepper and cook for about 1 minute or until fragrant. Add the prawns to the pan and cook for 2-3 minutes per side or until pink and fully cooked. Squeeze the lime juice over the prawns and mix well. Serve the spicy prawns with chilli sauce hot, garnished with chopped fresh parsley if preferred.

FRIED TOFU WITH VEGETABLES AND SOY SAUCE

Preparation Times: 15 minutes

Cooking Times: 10-15 minutes

Doses Ingredients for 4 People:

400g tofu, cut into cubes

2 tablespoons of olive oil

2 cloves garlic, finely chopped

1 red bell pepper, cut into thin strips

81 green pepper, cut into thin strips

1 carrot, cut into thin strips or julienne

1/2 cup broccoli, divided into small sprigs

1/4 cup soy sauce

1 tablespoon brown sugar

1 tablespoon cornstarch

Chopped fresh parsley for garnish (optional)

Preparation:

In a large skillet, heat the olive oil over medium-high heat. Add the cubed tofu and cook until golden on all sides. Remove tofu from pan and set aside. In the same pan, add the minced garlic and vegetables (peppers, carrot, broccoli) and cook for 5 to 7 minutes or until the vegetables are tender but still crunchy. Meanwhile, prepare the sauce by mixing the soy sauce, brown sugar and cornstarch in a bowl. Once the vegetables are cooked, add the tofu back to the pan and pour the sauce over the top. Cook for an additional 2-3 minutes or until the sauce has thickened slightly. Serve the stir-fried tofu with vegetables and hot soy sauce, garnished with chopped fresh parsley if desired.

CHICKEN PARMESAN WITH WHOLE WHOLE PASTA

Preparation Times: 20 minutes

Cooking Times: 30 minutes

Doses Ingredients for 4 People:

4 chicken breasts

Salt and black pepper to taste

1 cup flour

2 eggs, beaten

2 cups breadcrumbs

Olive oil for frying

1 cup marinara sauce

1 cup grated mozzarella

1/2 cup grated parmesan

300 g of wholemeal pasta

Chopped fresh parsley for garnish (optional)

Preparation:

Set up a breading station with three plates: one with flour, one with beaten eggs, and one with breadcrumbs. Season the chicken breasts with salt and black pepper, then dip them first in the flour, then in the beaten eggs and finally in the breadcrumbs. Heat the olive oil in a large skillet over medium-high heat and fry the chicken breasts until golden brown on both sides and fully cooked. Remove them from the pan and set aside. In a separate pot, cook whole-wheat pasta according to package instructions.

Drain the pasta. In a baking dish, add half of the marinara sauce. Arrange the fried chicken breasts on top of the sauce. Cover the chicken breasts with the rest of the marinara sauce, then sprinkle the grated mozzarella and grated parmesan on top. Bake in the preheated oven at 180°C for about 15 minutes or until the cheese is melted and golden. Serve the chicken parmigiana hot over whole-wheat pasta, garnished with fresh chopped parsley if you prefer.

BAKED PORK STEAK WITH SWEET POTATOES

Preparation Times: 15 minutes

Cooking Times: 35-40 minutes

Doses Ingredients for 4 People:

4 pork steaks

Salt and black pepper to taste

2 tablespoons of olive oil

2 sweet potatoes, peeled and sliced

1 onion, cut into slices

2 sprigs of fresh rosemary

2 tablespoons butter

Chopped fresh parsley

for garnish (optional)

Preparation:

Preheat the oven to 200°C. Season the pork steaks with salt and black pepper. In a large skillet, heat the olive oil over medium-high heat. Add the pork steaks and sear for 2-3 minutes per side or until browned. In a baking dish, arrange the sweet potato slices and onion slices. Place the pork steaks on top of the potatoes and onions. Add the rosemary sprigs and butter over the steaks. Cover the baking dish with foil and bake in the preheated oven for about 25 to 30 minutes or until the steaks are cooked through and the potatoes are tender. Serve the baked pork steaks with hot sweet potatoes, garnished with chopped fresh parsley if desired.

SALMON IN PAPER WITH BARLEY RISOTTO

Preparation Times: 20 minutes

Cooking Times: 20-25 minutes

Doses Ingredients for 4 People:

4 salmon fillets

Salt and black pepper to taste

2 cups of barley

1 onion, chopped

2 cloves garlic, finely chopped

4 cups hot fish or vegetable broth

1 cup dry white wine

1 lemon, thinly sliced

4 sheets of parchment paper or aluminum foil

Extra virgin olive oil

Chopped fresh parsley for garnish (optional)

Preparation:

Preheat the oven to 180°C. Season the salmon fillets with salt and black pepper. Place each fillet on a sheet of parchment paper or foil. In a saucepan, heat some olive oil and sauté the onion and garlic until golden. Add the barley to the pot and toast for a couple of minutes. Pour the white wine into the pan and let it evaporate. Add the hot fish or vegetable broth, a little at a time, stirring frequently and continuing to cook the barley until it is soft and creamy.

Place one salmon fillet on each sheet of parchment or foil. Spread the cooked barley next to the fillets. Add a few lemon slices on top of the salmon, then seal the parchment or foil packets tightly. Bake in the preheated oven for about 15-20 minutes or until the salmon is cooked through and flakes easily with a fork. Serve the salmon baked in foil with hot barley risotto, garnished with fresh chopped parsley if you prefer.

CHICKEN CACCIATORA WITH POLENTA

Preparation Times: 15 minutes

Cooking times: 1 hour

Doses Ingredients for 4 People:

4 chicken legs (thighs and thighs)

Salt and black pepper to taste

2 tablespoons of olive oil

1 onion, chopped

2 cloves garlic, finely chopped

1 red pepper, cut into strips

1 green pepper, cut into strips

1 courgette, cut into rounds

1 cup peeled tomatoes

1/2 cup red wine

1 tablespoon dried oregano

1 cup polenta flour

4 cups of water

Chopped fresh parsley for garnish (optional)

Preparation:

In a large pot, heat the olive oil over medium-high heat. Add the chicken thighs and brown until golden on all sides. Remove chicken from pot and set aside. In the same pot, add the onion, garlic, peppers and zucchini. Cook for 5 to 7 minutes or until vegetables are tender. Add the peeled tomatoes, red wine and oregano. Return chicken to pot.

Cover and cook over medium-low heat for about 45 minutes or until the chicken is cooked through and the sauce has thickened. Meanwhile, prepare the polenta by bringing water to a boil in a separate pot. Gradually, stir the polenta flour into the boiling water, stirring constantly until thick and creamy. If desired, add butter and grated parmesan to make the polenta even tastier. Serve the chicken Cacciatore hot over the polenta, garnished with fresh chopped parsley if you prefer.

TROUT FILLET WITH QUINOA AND VEGETABLES

Preparation Times: 15 minutes

Cooking Times: 20-25 minutes

Doses Ingredients for 4 People:

4 trout fillets

Salt and black pepper to taste

1 cup quinoa

2 cups water or vegetable broth

2 tablespoons of olive oil

1 red onion, thinly sliced

2 carrots, cut into thin rounds

1 courgette, cut into thin rounds

1 red pepper, cut into strips

Juice of 1 lemon

Preparation:

Preheat the oven to 180°C. Season the trout fillets with salt and black pepper. Place each fillet on foil or parchment paper. In a saucepan, bring water or vegetable broth to a boil. Add the quinoa and cook according to package instructions. Once cooked, set it aside. In a large skillet, heat the olive oil over medium heat. Add the red onion, carrots, zucchini and red bell pepper. Cook vegetables for 5 to 7 minutes or until tender but still crunchy. Squeeze the lemon juice over the vegetables. Layer the roasted vegetables over the trout fillets. Seal foil or parchment paper packets tightly. Bake in the preheated oven for about 15 minutes or until the fish is cooked through and flakes easily with a fork. Serve the trout fillet with quinoa and vegetables hot, garnished with fresh chopped parsley if you prefer.

BEEF STEAK WITH CAULIFLOWER PUREE

Preparation Times: 15 minutes

Cooking Times: 25-30 minutes

Doses Ingredients for 4 People:

4 beef steaks (200g each)

Salt and black pepper to taste

1 cauliflower, cut into florets

2 tablespoons butter

2 cloves garlic, finely chopped

1/2 cup milk

2 tablespoons grated parmesan

Chopped fresh parsley

for garnish (optional)

Preparation:

Bring a pan of lightly salted water to a boil. Add the cauliflower florets and cook for 10-12 minutes or until tender. Drain the cauliflower. In a skillet, heat the butter over medium-high heat. Add the minced garlic and cook for 1-2 minutes or until fragrant. Blend the cooked cauliflower with the garlic butter, milk, grated Parmesan, salt and black pepper until you have a creamy puree. Adjust the consistency with more milk if necessary. Season the beef steaks with salt and black pepper and cook on the grill or in a skillet over medium-high heat for 3 to 5 minutes per side or until done to your preferred doneness. Serve the sirloin steak with hot cauliflower puree, garnished with chopped fresh parsley if desired.

EGG OMELETATE WITH BACON AND POTATOES

Preparation Times: 15 minutes

Cooking Times: 20-25 minutes

Doses Ingredients for 4 People:

8 eggs

100g smoked bacon, diced

2 medium potatoes, peeled and cut into thin slices

1 onion, chopped

Salt and black pepper to taste

2 tablespoons of olive oil

Grated cheese to taste (optional)

Chopped fresh parsley

for garnish (optional)

Preparation:

Preheat the oven to 180°C. In a nonstick skillet, heat the olive oil over medium heat. Add the diced bacon and cook until crispy. Remove the bacon from the pan and set aside. In the same pan, add the potato slices and chopped onion. Cook until potatoes are golden and tender, about 10 to 12 minutes. Remove the potatoes and onion from the pan. In a bowl, beat the eggs and season them with salt and black pepper to taste. Pour the beaten eggs into the pan, then spread the crispy bacon, potatoes and onion evenly over the eggs.

Cook the omelette over medium-low heat for 5 to 7 minutes or until the edges begin to set. Transfer the pan to the preheated oven and cook the omelette for a further 8 to 10 minutes or until fully cooked and has a golden brown surface. Optionally, sprinkle the omelette with grated cheese and place it under the oven broiler for a couple of minutes to melt. Serve the omelette hot, garnished with fresh chopped parsley if you prefer.

CHICKEN CURRY WITH BROWN RICE

Preparation Times: 15 minutes

Cooking Times: 30-35 minutes

Doses Ingredients for 4 People:

4 chicken breasts, cut into cubes

Salt and black pepper to taste

2 tablespoons of olive oil

1 onion, chopped

2 cloves garlic, finely chopped

2 tablespoons curry paste (depending

desired level of spiciness)

1 can of coconut milk (400 ml)

2 tablespoons of tomato paste

2 cups brown rice, cooked

Chopped fresh parsley for garnish (optional)

Preparation:

In a large skillet, heat the olive oil over medium-high heat. Add the chicken cubes and cook until golden on all sides. Remove the chicken from the pan and set aside. In the same pan, add the chopped onion and minced garlic. Cook for 2-3 minutes until golden. Add the curry paste and cook for another minute, stirring well. Pour the coconut milk and tomato paste into the pan. Stir well to combine the ingredients. Return the chicken to the pan and cook over medium-low heat for 15 to 20 minutes or until the chicken is cooked through and the sauce is thickened. Serve the chicken curry over hot brown rice, garnished with chopped fresh parsley if desired.

FRENCH SOLE WITH MUSHROOM RISOTTO

Preparation Times: 20 minutes

Cooking Times: 30-35 minutes

Doses Ingredients for 4 People:

4 sole fillets

Salt and black pepper to taste

Flour for breading

2 eggs, beaten

2 tablespoons butter

2 tablespoons of olive oil

Juice of 1 lemon

1 cup Arborio rice

200g mixed mushrooms, cut into slices

1 onion, chopped

2 cloves garlic, finely chopped

1/2 cup dry white wine

4 cups hot chicken broth

2 tablespoons butter for the risotto

Grated parmesan cheese

for garnish (optional)

Chopped fresh parsley for

garnish (optional)

Preparation:

In a bowl, beat the eggs and season them with salt and pepper. Place the flour for the breading on a plate. Dip the sole fillets first in the flour, then in the beaten egg. In a large skillet, heat the butter and olive oil over medium-high heat. Cook the sole fillets until golden on both sides, about 2-3 minutes per side. Squeeze the lemon juice over the fillets and set aside.

In the same pan, add the chopped onion and garlic. Cook for 2-3 minutes until golden. Add the Arborio rice and chopped mushrooms and cook for another minute, stirring well. Pour the white wine into the pan and cook until it has evaporated. Begin adding the chicken broth one ladleful at a time, stirring constantly and waiting for the liquid to be absorbed before adding more. Continue this process until the risotto is creamy and the rice is cooked (about 18-20 minutes). Stir the butter into the risotto and season with salt and black pepper to taste. Serve the French sole over the mushroom risotto, garnished with grated parmesan and chopped fresh parsley if preferred.

MUSTARD PORK WITH CARROT PURE

Preparation Times: 15 minutes

Cooking Times: 25-30 minutes

Doses Ingredients for 4 People:

4 pork steaks

Salt and black pepper to taste

2 tablespoons Dijon mustard

2 tablespoons of olive oil

4 medium carrots, peeled and cut into slices

2 medium potatoes, peeled and cut into cubes

2 tablespoons butter

1/2 cup milk

Chopped fresh parsley

for garnish (optional)

Preparation:

Preheat the oven to 180°C. Season pork steaks with salt, black pepper, and Dijon mustard on both sides. In a large skillet, heat the olive oil over medium-high heat. Cook pork steaks until browned on both sides, about 3 to 4 minutes per side. Transfer the pork steaks to a baking sheet and cook in the preheated oven for 15 to 20 minutes or until cooked through and have reached the desired internal temperature. Meanwhile, bring a pot of salted water to a boil. Add the carrots and potatoes and cook until tender, about 15 to 20 minutes. Drain them. Mash the carrots and potatoes with a pestle or fork. Add the butter and milk and mix until you get a creamy consistency. Season with salt and black pepper to taste. Serve the mustard pork steaks with the warm carrot puree, garnished with chopped fresh parsley if desired.

PRAWNS IN COCONUT CREAM WITH ZOODLES

Preparation Times: 15 minutes

Cooking Times: 15-20 minutes

Doses Ingredients for 4 People:

500 g of peeled and cleaned prawns

Salt and black pepper to taste

2 tablespoons of olive oil

1 red onion, chopped

2 cloves garlic, finely chopped

1 fresh red chili pepper, chopped (optional)

1 can of coconut milk (400 ml)

1 lemon, juice and zest

4 courgettes, made into zoodles

(cut into julienne strips like spaghetti)

Chopped fresh parsley for garnish (optional)

Preparation:

In a large skillet, heat the olive oil over medium-high heat. Add the chopped onion, garlic and chilli (if using) and cook for 2-3 minutes until golden. Add the shrimp to the pan and cook for 3 to 4 minutes or until pink and set. Remove the shrimp from the pan and set aside. In the same pan, pour the coconut milk, lemon juice and zest.

Mix well and cook over medium heat for 5-7 minutes or until the sauce thickens slightly. Add the shrimp to the coconut sauce and cook for another 2-3 minutes. Season with salt and black pepper to taste. Meanwhile, prepare zoodles with a spiralizer or vegetable peeler to create thin zucchini strips. Serve the shrimp and coconut cream over the courgette zoodles, garnishing with chopped fresh parsley if desired.

PULLED PORK WITH CALES SALAD

Preparation Times: 15 minutes

Cooking times: 3 hours

(in the oven at low temperature)

Doses Ingredients for 4 People:

1kg pork (shoulder or loin) cut into pieces

Salt and black pepper to taste

2 tablespoons of olive oil

1 onion, chopped

3 cloves garlic, finely chopped

1 cup chicken broth

1/2 cup barbecue sauce

1/4 cup apple cider vinegar

1 tablespoon brown sugar

1 teaspoon smoked paprika (optional)

4 hamburger or brioche buns

960 g. of green cabbage, thinly sliced

1 carrot, grated

1/2 cup mayonnaise

2 tablespoons red wine vinegar

Salt and black pepper to taste

Preparation:

Preheat the oven to 350°F if you plan to cook the pork in the oven. Season the pork with salt and black pepper. In a large skillet, heat the olive oil over medium-high heat. Add the pork and brown on all sides until browned. Transfer the pork to a slow cooker (if using) or baking dish (if cooking in the oven). In the same pan, add the chopped onion and garlic.

Cook for 2-3 minutes until golden. Add the chicken broth, barbecue sauce, apple cider vinegar, brown sugar, and smoked paprika (if using). Bring everything to a boil, then pour it over the pork. Cook the pork in the oven, cover the baking dish with foil, and cook for 3 to 4 hours or until tender. While the pork cooks, prepare the coleslaw. In a large bowl, mix the cabbage, carrot, mayonnaise, red wine vinegar, salt, and black pepper to taste. Set aside. Once cooked, shred the pork with a fork until it has a pulled consistency. Serve pulled pork on hamburger or brioche buns, accompanied by fresh coleslaw.

SESAME CHICKEN WITH STEAMED BROCCOLI

Preparation Times: 15 minutes

Cooking Times: 15-20 minutes

Doses Ingredients for 4 People:

4 skinless chicken breasts

Salt and black pepper to taste

2 tablespoons sesame seeds

2 tablespoons sesame oil

2 tablespoons soy sauce

1 tablespoon honey

2 cloves garlic, finely chopped

4 cups broccoli, cut into florets

1 tablespoon olive oil

Preparation:

Preheat the oven to 200°C. Season the chicken breasts with salt, black pepper and sesame seeds. In a large nonstick skillet, heat the sesame oil over medium-high heat. Add the chicken and cook for 2-3 minutes per side until golden. In a bowl, mix the soy sauce, honey and minced garlic. Pour this mixture over the chicken in the pan. Transfer the pan to the preheated oven and cook for 10 to 12 minutes or until the chicken is cooked through and the juices run clear when pierced with a fork. Meanwhile, bring a pan of lightly salted water to a boil. Add the broccoli and steam for 3-4 minutes or until tender but crisp. Drain them and season them with a little olive oil, salt and black pepper. Serve the sesame chicken with the steamed broccoli.

GRILLED SALMON WITH ALMOND BUTTER SAUCE

Preparation Times: 10 minutes

Cooking Times: 10-15 minutes

Doses Ingredients for 4 People:

4 salmon fillets

Salt and black pepper to taste

2 tablespoons of olive oil

1 cup toasted almonds

4 tablespoons butter

Juice of 1 lemon

Chopped fresh parsley

for garnish (optional)

Preparation:

Preheat grill to medium-high heat. Season the salmon fillets with salt, black pepper and olive oil. In a skillet, melt the butter over medium heat. Add the toasted almonds and cook for 2-3 minutes until the butter is golden brown. Add the lemon juice to the butter sauce and mix well. Grill the salmon fillets for 4-5 minutes per side or until cooked to desired doneness. Pour the almond butter sauce over the grilled salmon and garnish with chopped fresh parsley if desired.

GRILLED TUNA WITH AVOCADO SAUCE

Preparation Times: 15 minutes

Cooking Times: 5-7 minutes

Doses Ingredients for 4 People:

4 fresh tuna fillets

Salt and black pepper to taste

2 tablespoons of olive oil

For the avocado salsa:

2 ripe avocados, peeled

and deprived of the stone

Juice of 1 lime

2 tablespoons chopped fresh coriander

Salt and black pepper to taste

Preparation:

Preheat grill to medium-high heat. Season the tuna fillets with salt, black pepper and olive oil. Grill the tuna for 2-3 minutes per side or until cooked to desired doneness. Tuna can be served slightly pink in the center. Meanwhile, prepare the avocado salsa. In a bowl, mash the avocado pulp with a fork. Add lime juice, chopped fresh cilantro, salt and black pepper. Mix well until you get a creamy sauce. Serve the grilled tuna with the avocado sauce on top.

CONCLUSION

Thank you for taking your time to read this book on the Carb Cycling Diet for Beginners. I hope you found the information useful and that it helps you achieve your health and fitness goals. The journey to a fit and healthy body is unique to each of us, and I am honored to have been able to share with you an approach that can make a real difference in your life. If you found this book useful, I invite you to leave a review. Your feedback is extremely valuable, not only to me, but also to other readers who may benefit from this information. A positive review can help this book reach more people, supporting them on their journey to a healthier life. Finally, I want to express my sincere gratitude for choosing to read this book. Your commitment to improving your health and well-being is truly admirable, and I hope this book has helped you on your journey. I wish you the better for the future and I thank you once again for sharing part of your journey with me. --- This conclusion creates a personal connection with readers, expressing gratitude and encouraging them to leave a review in a kind and positive way. So, we conclude this book with an invitation: be the protagonist of your health, experience Carb Cycling responsibly and enjoy the results that come from it. May 2024 be the year you start living your life to the fullest, with energy, vitality and confidence. Happy journey to a new and better version of yourself! Thank you for choosing "Carb Cycling Diet 2024" as your guide. May you be successful on your path to optimal health and wellness! Love, [TERY LONG]

www.ingramcontent.com/pod-product-compliance
Lightning Source LLC
Chambersburg PA
CBHW070649250726
48662CB00001B/37